Breaking the Food Chain

A Simple Guide to Better Health

Jack Chou

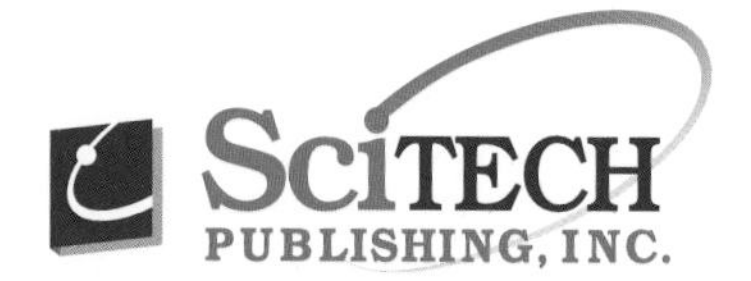

Product Development: Cathy Gileadi Wilson
Illustrations: Paul Kuo
Photography: Jack Chou
Page Composition and Cover Design: Shyam Reyes
Copy Editing and Proofreading: Julie Sartain

Printed by Overseas Printing Corporation

©2002 by Jack Chou. All rights reserved. No part of this book may be reproduced or used in any form whatsoever without the written permission from the publisher except in the case of brief quotations embodied in critical articles and reviews. For information, contact the publisher, SciTech Publishing, 5601 N. Hawthorne Way, Raleigh, NC 27613.

Printed in Korea

10 9 8 7 6 5 4 3 2 1

ISBN 1-891121-18-9

For ordering information:
SciTech Publishing, Inc.
5601 N. Hawthorne Way
Raleigh, NC 27613
(919) 866-1501
orders@scitechpub.com
http://www.scitechpub.com

This book is available in bulk quantities at discount for special premium use by contacting the SciTech Publishing Special Sales Dept.

TABLE OF CONTENTS

About the Author

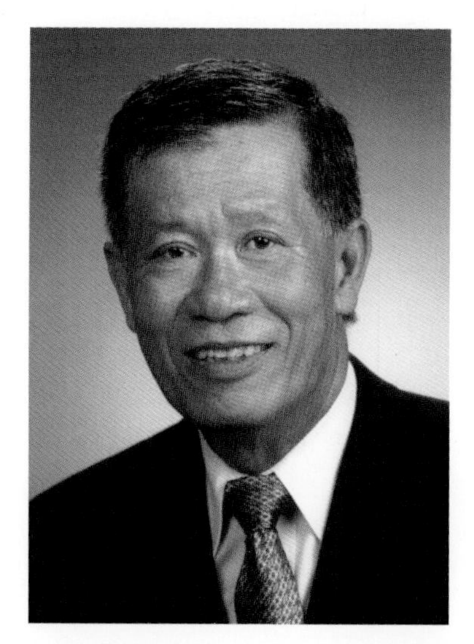

Jack Chou was born in Taiwan during the Japanese occupation (Japan occupied Taiwan from 1895 to the end of World War II, 1945).

During World War II, his family experienced air raids and daily bombings by the American bombers because Taiwan was a Japanese possession. After the war, the Nationalist Chinese took over Taiwan, at the time losing their battle fighting the Communists on the Chinese mainland. The innocent Taiwanese got caught on the wrong side of both military conflicts. Consequently, while growing up, Jack experienced many economic and personal hardships, especially a shortage of food. Today, these wartime experiences are still vivid in his memory and play an important role in his respect for food and his daily appreciation of the food we eat.

In 1962, Jack arrived in America as a student. Along with many young immigrants to America, he used a student visa to escape from the political turmoil and pessimism in Taiwan, leaving it all behind to seek new opportunities in this promised land. He graduated with a Master's degree in Mechanical Engineering from Southern Methodist University in Dallas, Texas. After graduation, Jack worked briefly as an aerospace engineer. Through research into a field that interested him, Jack started a company manufacturing instruments that protect against toxic and combustible gas.

That was almost thirty years ago. Jack's qualifications to write this book are not based on his professional training or experience as a nutritionist or medical doctor, but rather on his conclusions as a trained scientist. Jack has a natural disposition and aptitude for analyzing problems, researching their underlying causes, and seeking practical solutions. Just to survive, growing up during Japanese Imperial and Chinese Autocratic regimes, Jack learned to be very skeptical (and suspicious) of any establishment propaganda. In the process, he learned to make detailed analyses of any issues, and to decide for himself how best to proceed. Jack's unique experience with Japanese and Chinese cultures has enabled him to observe the American way of life from a different perspective than that of a typical American. All of these experiences have led to this book, which we think will help many Americans lead a healthier life.

About Paul Kuo and the Formosan Vignette

The numerous watercolors and sketches throughout this book are all the work of my friend Paul Kuo. The watercolor paintings were specifically created for this book while the sketches were selected from the "*Formosan Vignette*," also by Paul, which originally appeared in the Taiwan-English newspaper in the late 1950s and early 1960s.

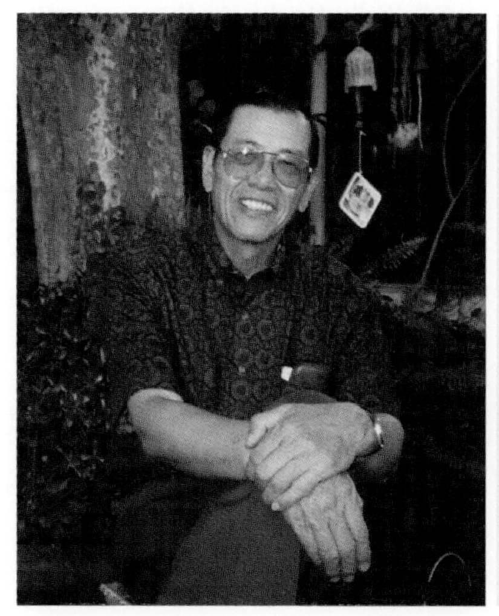

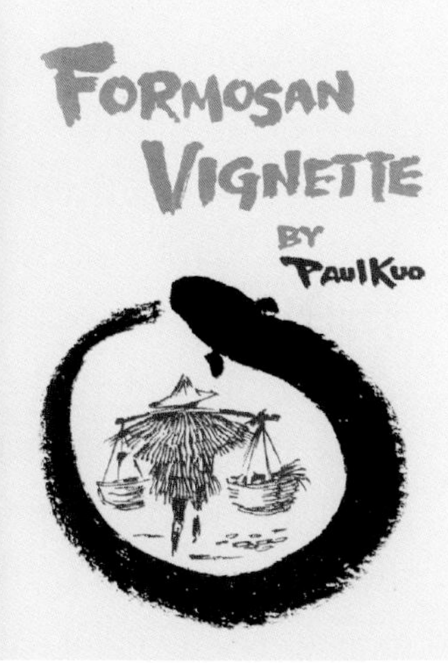

Paul was born of Taiwanese parents in Tokyo, Japan. As a student at Taiwan University, majoring in languages in the late fifties, Paul was affiliated with the China Post, the only English-language newspaper at that time in Taiwan. He contributed a column known as the *Formosan Vignette* for many years. After World War II, and the Korean War, there were numerous American newcomers to Taiwan. The Taiwanese customs and everyday aspects of daily Taiwanese life were interesting to the newly arrived, curious American visitors. In the form of pen and ink sketches, Paul cast his observant eye over the land and people of Taiwan. His artistic and illustrative skill built a bridge for Americans to understand the Taiwanese culture and life.

Paul and I met while serving our compulsory military training for officers after graduation from college. At over six feet, he was the tallest of the full company of 132 men, and being slightly shorter than him, I was number two. As fervent Taiwanese patriots, we immediately became good friends. Paul's *Formosan Vignette* drawings were gathered into a book in the 1960s. While reviewing his book, I recalled that there were many nostalgic, interesting illustrations of the Taiwanese way of life in the *Formosan Vignette*. It also depicted the healthy life style of yesteryear before the intrusion of technology. As you read this book, I hope you will agree that Paul's art has contributed much to this book.

Paul currently resides in Scottsdale, Arizona, and has studios both in Scottsdale and Taipei. In his own words about his painting: "Most of my watercolors grow out of quick outdoor sketches. Instead of finishing them right on the spot, I take them to my studio and use nature as a starting point for the final painting. I usually wet the entire surface of the paper using a sponge, as watercolor pigment spreads better while it is wet."

As a late member of the Board of Trustees of the Phoenix Art Museum, Dr. William S. Shields, wrote: "Paul is one of our most exciting contemporary watercolorists. He is one of the few outstanding watercolor artists painting Indian and Southwestern subjects. His paintings capture the picturesque charm of people and landscapes of Canyon de Chelly, Monument Valley and the Taos pueblo. . ."

Among other exhibits, every other year, Paul has a major exhibit in Alhambra, California, near Los Angeles.

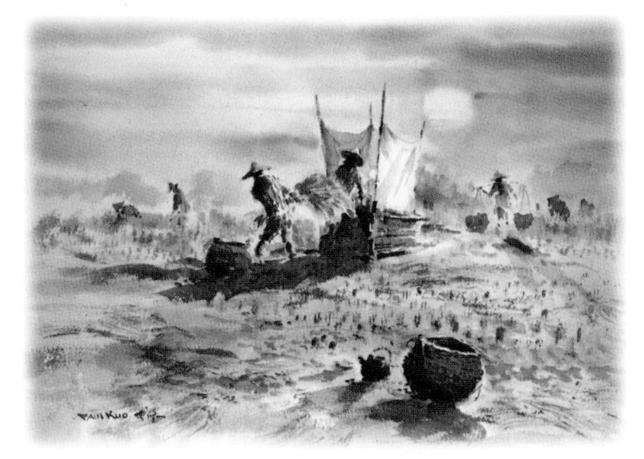

"HARVEST" watercolor by Paul Kuo

"...my thoughts draw from the old traditions of cultures that valued balance and common sense."

A Guide to the Reader

I believe that every American can adopt a better and more enjoyable eating plan that will improve health and enhance the eating experience. Not based on calories and the "diets" prescribed by doctors with a "lose weight fast" scheme, my thoughts draw from the old traditions of cultures that valued balance and common sense. I will show you how the British and European traditions have melded with modern food processing and fast-food advertising to take us off the track of a healthy diet. Most of this information is derived from my Taiwanese roots, which you can readily identify with the wisdom of your own parents or grandparents.

The foods that you are already familiar with can be enhanced with painless, and even enjoyable, cooking and preparation techniques. You may also learn about some new foods that are easily obtained and delicious. More than a cookbook or diet book, this book is designed to be a thought-provoking tour through the landscape of American eating habits and the often neglected side roads that reveal the beauty and enjoyments of a simpler, more rewarding approach to one of life's pleasures.

I hope that you will enjoy reading this book, learn some fascinating things about food and your body, and that it will empower you to adapt your lifestyle to a new way of eating and living that can bring you good health for the rest of a long life.

— Jack Chou, *Irvine, California*

Acknowledgments

For a professional engineer and scientist, without any formal training in nutritional science, to compose a book like this, I required the assistance and suggestions from many sources.

Special thanks to Cathy Gileadi Wilson, herbalist, healer, mother of nine, and author of the book *Simple and Essential*. With her outstanding writing skills and knowledge about food and health, she not only contributed to the writing of this book but also offered many valuable ideas and suggestions.

Copy-editing and proofreading, as well as additional suggestions for improvement to this work were provided by Julie Sartain, writer, editor, artist, and computer scientist. The power of the Internet made all of this possible. Both Cathy and Julie reside near Salt Lake City, Utah, and we finished the project just as if we were all in the same office.

I was also fortunate to have the extensive advice and mentoring of Dudley Kay, writer, editor, and founder and president of SciTech Publishing, who published my first book, *Hazardous Gas Monitors*.

And special thanks to my brother-in-law John Schoepf, an environmental consultant who grew up in a small farming community in central California, who helped me compare the American lifestyle with my Taiwan experiences, which inspired many ideas for this book.

The creative arrangement and interesting presentation is the work of Shyam Reyes, artist, Webmaster, and musician, and I thank him for his outstanding artistic page layout and book design.

And last, there are no words to express my gratitude to my life-long friend Paul Kuo for his contribution of the watercolors specifically painted for the purpose of the book, and his interesting cartoon-like line drawings depicting life and customs of the Taiwanese. His work adds a color and quality to this book that would be lost without his art.

Finally, I want to express my gratitude to my family, including my sons, David, Daniel and Thomas, who gave me much advice and assistance; my daughter-in-law Charlotte, who spent numerous hours proofreading and editing; and my wife Doris, whose constant encouragement was invaluable.

PART ONE

Setting the Table: Why We Eat What We Eat

Science and technology have improved our lives, while at the same time making our daily living even more complex and hectic. In the face of information overload, or indecipherable scientific studies, we are often left with little choice but to place our trust in the "professionals" who interpret and apply this esoteric knowledge to many areas of our daily lifestyles. But if the 1960s generation cautioned their contemporaries to "Question authority!" in a political context, now is a good time for this senior citizen, in this new millennium, to remind you of this maxim in the face of all that science and technology seem to promise us in regard to diet and nutrition.

To understand why and how the American diet is as it is today, I find it not only necessary but also interesting to trace the American diet back to its origins in British cooking. Even if we do not all have ancestors from Merry Olde England, we are, nonetheless, affected by the English influence carried over by the first colonists. It was they who established our food traditions from a limited menu of food choices and preparation techniques.

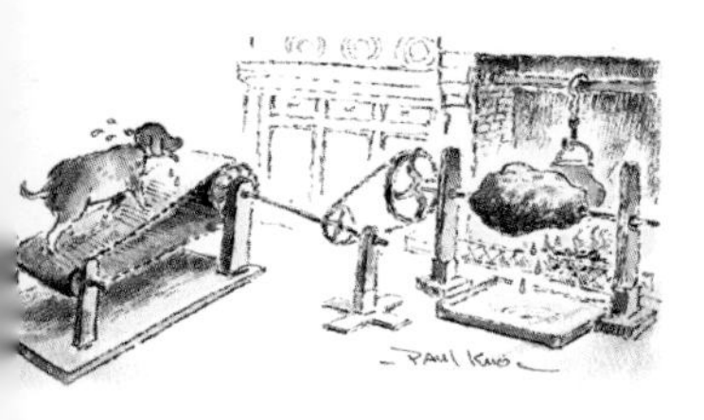

In **Chapter One** we discover how our diet today remains primarily British, modified by the lifestyle changes that have evolved from the industrial/technological revolution. My good artist friend Paul Kuo has contributed an illustrative watercolor to this chapter, and throughout the subsequent chapters, that I think you will find an eye-pleasing enhancement to the central points of the book.

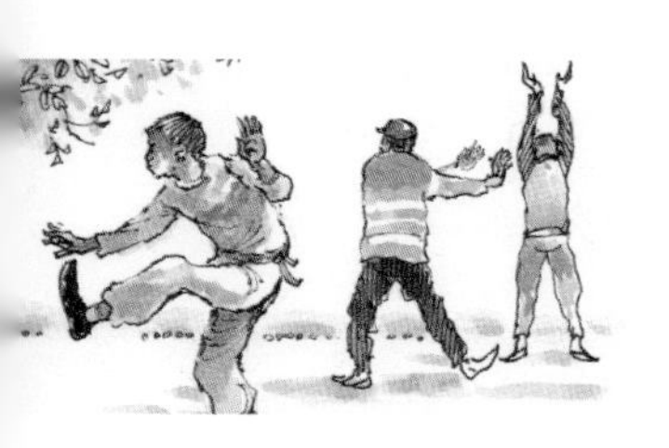

In **Chapter Two** we discuss how technology has changed the very nature of our food and how the alteration in readily available, tasty, and beautifully packaged food has seduced us into believing that our bodies can be treated as mechanical devices. We nearly all are cursed with what I have termed a resulting 'Shrimp Mentality.' You'll learn what I mean by this term as you read further.

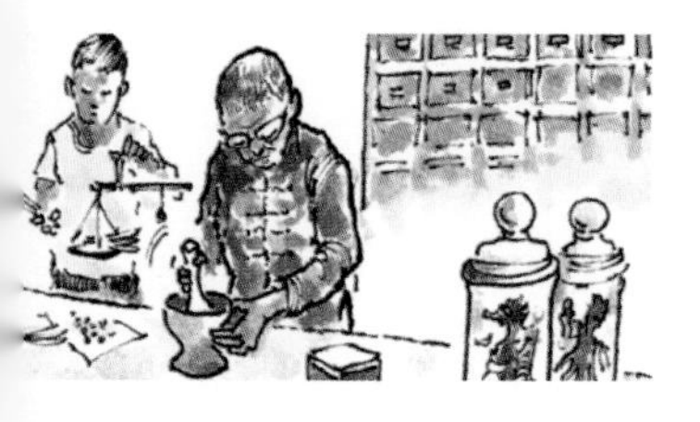

In **Chapter Three** we look at the old wisdom of East and West and take advantage of the best of the Old and New worlds. America's most famous humorist, Mark Twain, once observed that the older he grew, the smarter his father became. So maybe we, too, can learn from ancestors and older traditions that may have been dismissed as ignorant or old-fashioned.

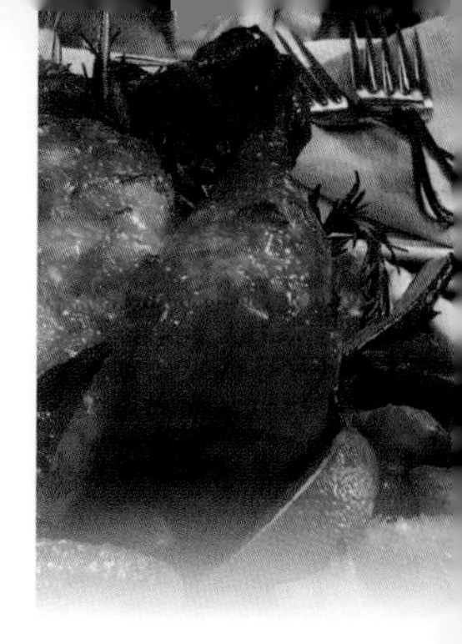

Chapter 1

English Cooking: Root of the American Diet

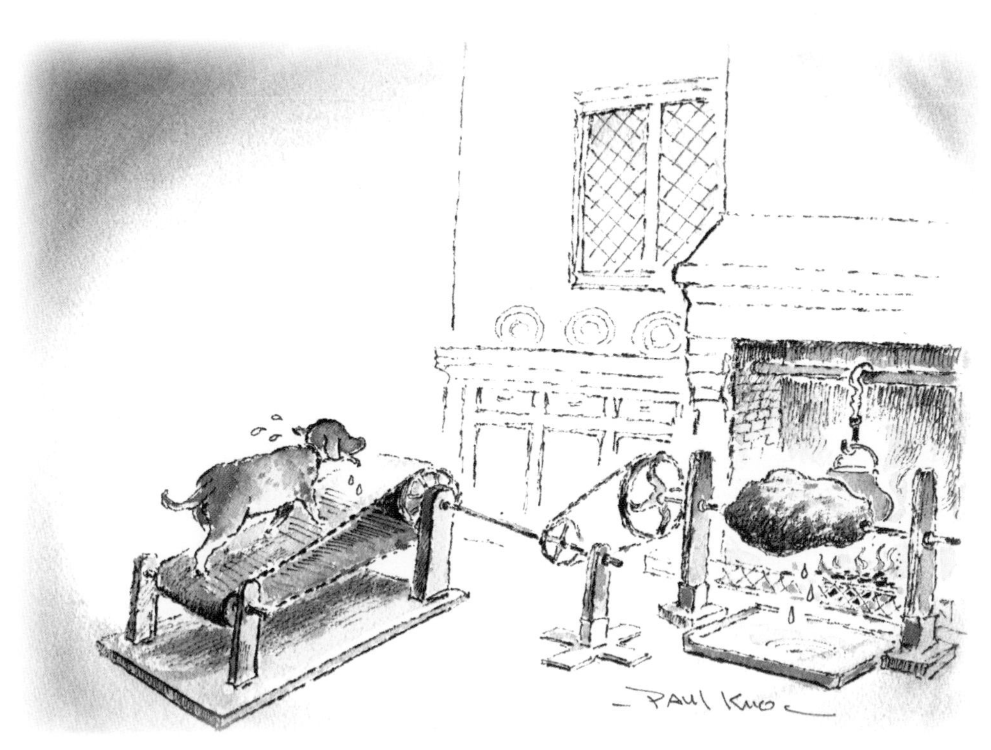

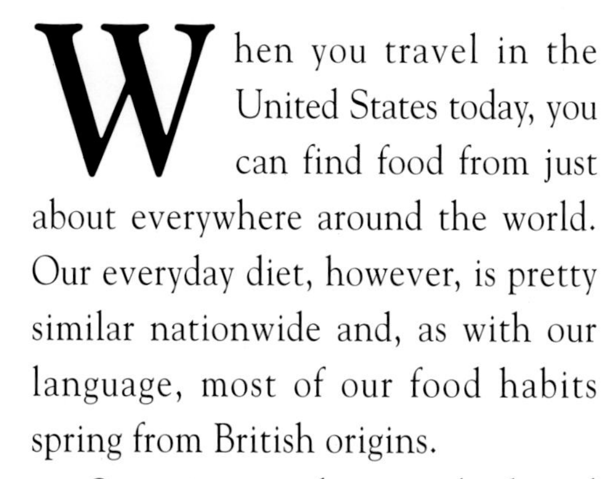

When you travel in the United States today, you can find food from just about everywhere around the world. Our everyday diet, however, is pretty similar nationwide and, as with our language, most of our food habits spring from British origins.

Over time, cooking methods and ingredients have evolved and changed, but the basic framework remains British. If we want to understand why we eat as we do, we need to look at how the British ate in the past.

Early English Foods

Like any indigenous culture in early England, people ate what was around them, what they could gather or grow in their surroundings. Diet varied from place to place, but people ate pretty much the same. They supplied their main protein by hunting and fishing—hunting during the winter and fishing during the summer. To keep meat between seasons, the British learned to preserve it by smoking, salting, drying, and curing with honey or sugar.

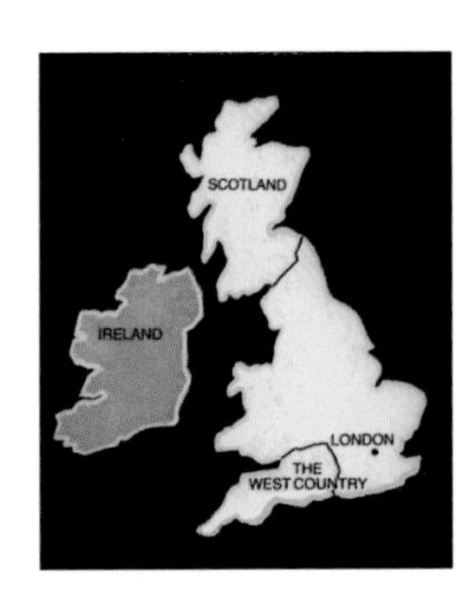

England, we may need to remind ourselves, is an island, so the people ate a considerable amount of fish, including whale, cod, ling, haddock, herring, and anchovies. Oddly enough, sea birds such as puffins and even geese were considered 'fish' and eaten as well.

When the Roman armies invaded England, they introduced the Greco-Roman ways of preparing food, so the British began pot-cooking their fish with herbs such as parsley, sage, rosemary, dittany, thyme, garlic, and pepper and adding condiments such as salt, vinegar, and ale.

They also baked fish into pies, eaten both hot and cold. The pastry, or shell of the pie, was viewed as a 'coffin' for cooking the fish—not always consumed with it. The English also cooked their fish into stews, hash, and bisque. Typically, braised or steamed fish was served with a sauce made of parsley chopped into melted butter and slightly thickened with flour.

Fast Days and Fish

In addition to cookery, the Romans introduced their form of Christianity to Britain, which included fast days such as Lent. The Church—or the King—imposed fast days to conserve the country's meat supply, though ostensibly for religious reasons. The fast was intended to make people more spiritual by mortifying the flesh and removing the pleasure of eating meat, which would reduce carnal passions thought to be inflamed by too-meaty a diet.

If an individual was sick, he could get a license from the priest permitting him to eat meat during the fast— a period that could last for months at a time. Interestingly, the British didn't class fish with meat, so you could eat fish and sea birds during a fast. For this reason, fish was considered an inferior and less desirable food in this tradition. People evidently didn't enjoy eating fish in the same way as meat, and eating too much fish was considered

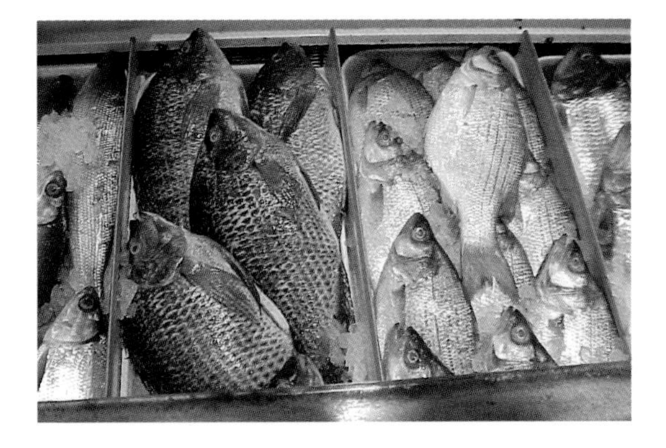

unwholesome, contrary to the medical opinions of today.

English Love of Meat

Where did the early British get their meat? Mostly from hunting in the rich forests, which provided abundant game such as deer, rabbits, and wild pigs. By the seventeenth century, the creation of large country estates allowed landowners to enclose what was formerly common land to grow meat animals more easily. This naturally led to experiments in breeding better meat animals. For example, during the eighteenth century, wild pigs were crossbred with imported Chinese pigs, which dramatically improved the quality of the pork. Before long, domestic meat replaced wild meat on most British tables.

The English consumed vast quantities of meat—enough to evoke comments from guests from other countries. In the 1690s, a European visitor named Mr. M. Mission, wrote: " . . . the English were great flesh eaters, and I found it true. I have known people in England that never eat any bread, and universally, they eat very little: they nibble a few crumbs while they chew the meat by whole mouthfuls."

"Among the middling sort of people, they have ten or twelve sorts of common meats which infallibly take their turns at

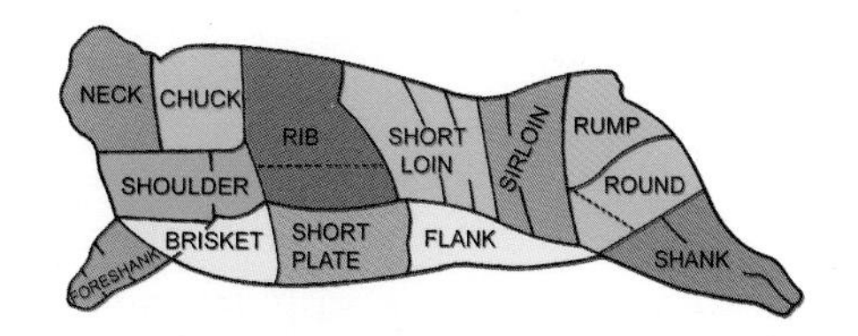

the tables, and two dishes are their dinners: a pudding, for instance, and a piece of roast beef. I do not believe that any Englishman who is his own master has ever eaten a dinner without meat." He also observed that the English dressed their meat plain and cooked simply with little seasoning.

Spit Roasting

The favorite British meat dish was spit-roasted. In early times, a turnspit boy turned the meat; in Tudor times, the turnspit dog replaced him. A small dog was trained to run continuously on a treadmill or in a circular cage to turn the spit, which was linked via a pulley system to the spit.

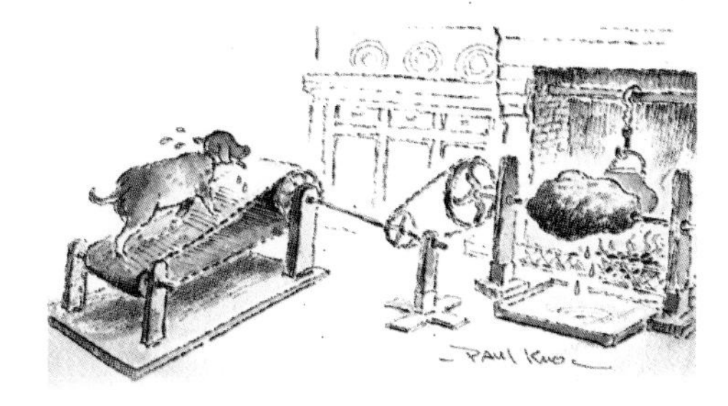

As the engineering knowledge improved, a mechanical gravity device became available. It functioned like an oversized, mechanical clock. A heavy weight was hung at one end of the rope, the rope was wound around a shaft, and as the weight descended, the mechanism rotated the spit. Like a grandfather's clock, it needed to be rewound.

English roasts are particularly remarkable for two things. First, English meat has a savory, delicious taste, perhaps because of the excellent pasture where the animals are raised. If you have traveled in England, you have seen the most beautifully cultivated meadows, which produce nourishing and sweet-scented hay. Second, nobody in the world understands the art of roasting meat like the English.

Raising beef cattle resulted in an increase of dairy products. Housewives turned these products into butter and cheese, which kept better than fresh milk, necessary prior to refrigeration. Most people consumed a lot of butter; it was used in almost every recipe: for cakes and pastry, to fry fish, to baste meat, in pottage and porridge, and buttered ales. It was also added to boiled food, either as it cooked or else melted over the dish at serving time, just as we use it today. So roasted meat and generous amounts of butter were common elements of the British diet.

Porridge - Food for the Poor, Healthy for All

You may be familiar with the term *porridge*, as in cooked cereal (usually oatmeal in England), but perhaps not so familiar with *pottage*. Pottage originated from the French term, 'potage,' which means soup. Pottage might include any combination of vegetables, grains, meat, or fish. The poorer people ate more grains because they could not afford much meat. Pottage might also include native plants such as leeks, garlic, roots of all kinds, nettle greens, etc., and be made of barley, oats, wheat, and rye, plus all kinds of meat, including fish.

Pottage became "porridge" when it contained only cereals, usually a breakfast food like it is today. Grains were ground and then cooked in water until soft and thick—a food for the poor man who could not afford much meat. Based on our knowledge about foods today, this poor man's rations contained well-balanced nutrients. It was also easy to digest and very hearty and satisfying.

Well-prepared porridge is an ideal dish to complement our over-rich diet, especially for individuals who want to lose a few pounds. See Chapter 11 for some ideas regarding how to make hearty, delicious porridge.

Potatoes and White Bread

For many years, the British relied on grains for their carbohydrates. In the late sixteenth century, the potato was introduced into England. It took some time for the British to develop a taste for potatoes, but by the eighteenth century, potatoes

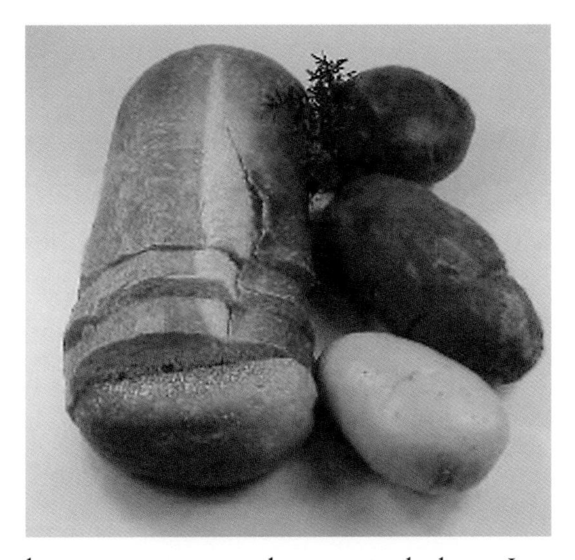

became quite popular, particularly in Ireland. Not only were potatoes easier to grow than oats or barley, they were safer. In an era of turbulence and uprisings when the military practiced a scorched-earth policy, an underground crop of potatoes was harder to find and destroy than a crop of grain. By the early eighteenth century, each time there was a poor cereal harvest, potatoes became more and more popular.

Nevertheless, bread was still a staple food. The British used all manner of grains and legumes: wheat, rye, barley, beans, peas, oats, and even acorns. Before the production of consistent, commercial yeasts, many bakers and housewives made fermented breads such as sourdough. These are now considered more digestible than plain-yeasted breads.

Traditionally, people preferred white bread made of wheat, not only for its light color and pleasant flavor, but because they believed it was easier to digest than other grainy, dry, or coarse breads. It was more expensive to make because the bran and germ had to be removed by roller polishing. We know now that this process also removes many valuable nutrients. Nevertheless, white bread remains popular to this day. In those days, the bakers secretly used artificial colors and bleaches to create a whiter loaf, another practice that continues to this day—only not as secretly.

In 1760, a British lord named John Montague, fourth Earl of Sandwich, wanted to keep gambling at his gaming table so, as legend has it, he ordered his meat served at the gaming table on bread, which created the first sandwich and resulted in its name, perhaps the most popular use of bread everywhere.

High Life Tradition

Americans adopted the British love of meat, and the way we eat meat today is very much in the old English style. Seafood has gained in popularity, but only in recent years after the health benefits of fish became known and preparation techniques significantly improved. But many still don't care for seafood much. Most cultures consider vegetables to be very healthy foods. However, in England, they aren't as prominent in everyday cooking, and British cooks typically don't prepare them very well. In this country, we have inherited the British methods of preparing vegetables with predictable results. Maybe that's why many Americans, especially children, have an aversion to vegetables. Without the balance provided by fish and vegetables, the British diet of meat, butter, and potatoes became the rather unwholesome norm for the well-to-do.

Early American Food

So what happened when the British settlers came to America? More than 95 percent of the population lived as farmers, quite different from America today. Like their British relatives, they raised, butchered, and cured their own meats, and they ate a lot of meat. Salt pork was the most important meat because pigs were easy to raise, they ate a variety of feeds, and they matured rapidly. People salted down the pork to keep for winter use.

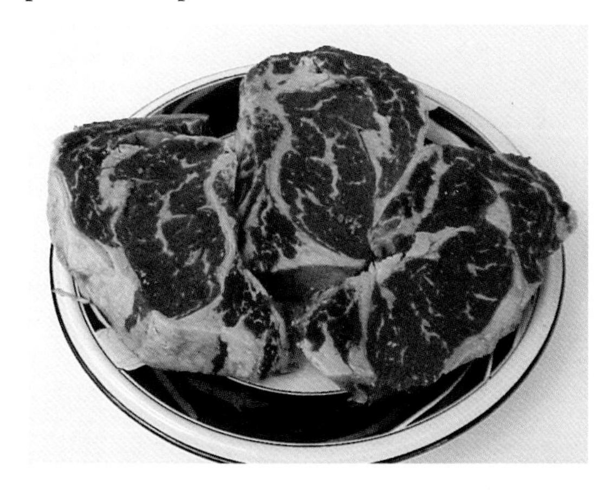

Beef was popular, but it wasn't eaten as commonly as it is today because beef was more expensive. In addition, most Americans supplemented their protein with game hunted from the surrounding forests such as squirrel, deer, wild ducks, and geese. They harvested garden produce and grains as well. There are few isolated communities left in the United States today that live in such a self-sufficient way, but in colonial times, the only food you could get was what you grew, gathered, or hunted.

Early Americans had three meals a day: breakfast, dinner, and supper, just as they dined back in the old country. Breakfast was light and often consisted of grain porridge or leftovers from the previous day. Dinner, the midday meal, was the largest and most important meal of the day. Supper was also a light meal and consisted primarily of food left over from the dinner table.

Because cooking was difficult and time-consuming, just as it was in England, most people cooked one large—or we could even say enormous—meal a day, planning to eat leftovers at supper and breakfast. We still eat this way on holidays like Thanksgiving and Christmas, probably out of tradition.

Living Off the Land

Pre-industrialized American cuisine remained very British in nature. But despite the similarities to British cuisine, the American diet was unique almost from the beginning, which is logical, considering that local foods were different in America. Many families relied on cornbread made from Native American corn as a daily staple. In addition, as they acclimated to the new land, they depended more and more on native foods such as pumpkins, squash, beans, and wild turkey.

Because America is so much closer to the Caribbean Islands than it is to the Far East, people soon substituted coffee for tea and rum for the European whiskey. Most early Americans didn't like the bitter taste of coffee, so they added generous amounts of sugar and cream.

Compared to what we eat today, that early diet seems very bland and monotonous with dishes largely based on the same components day after day, which is to be expected since people only had a limited variety of foods available.

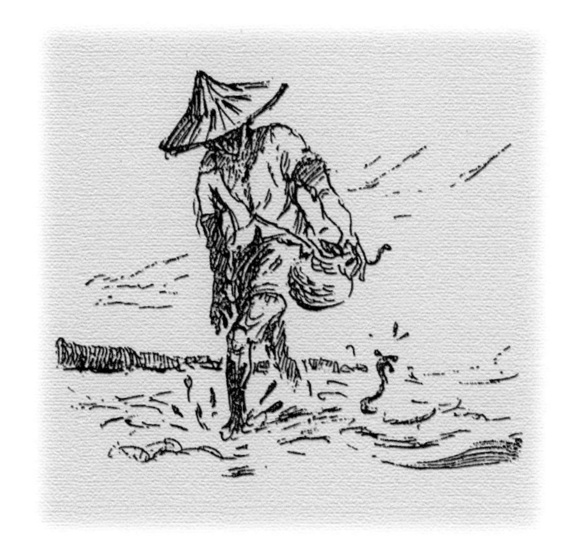

"Snakes" in the paddy. When the harvest is all complete and things have stagnated for a month or so, it is time for the farmers to catch the paddy eels. They trample over the muddy fields, and the slippery critters obligingly jump up to be caught.

Effects of the Industrial Revolution

The industrial revolution offered a great change to all of that, but the American diet has still remained very close to its cultural roots. It is human nature to enjoy foods that are familiar. Most people have a difficult time giving up familiar foods and accepting new tastes and textures, although in present-day America, more people are willing to branch out and try new things.

With the industrial revolution came a new lifestyle. People moved from working their farms to factory employment, which meant that large numbers of people worked far from home so they had to have their mid-day meal—formerly the large one—away from home.

This fundamentally changed the eating habits of the American population. Lunch began to replace dinner as a lighter meal. Starting with the necessity of changing schedules for factory workers, Americans began to eat a more substantial and

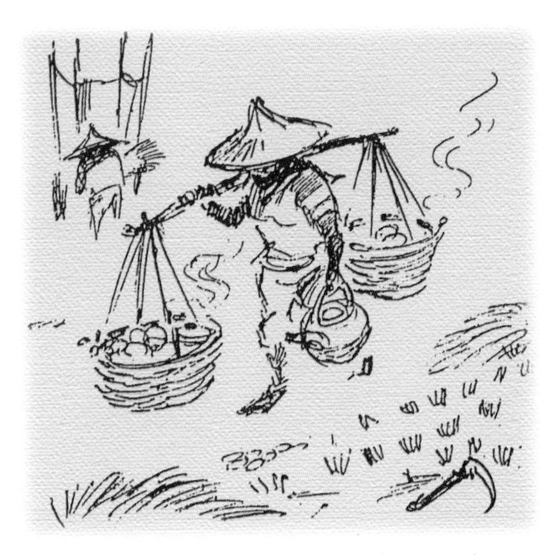

Harvest meals. In Taiwan, the rice harvesting begins in early summer and lasts until late autumn. The workman is worthy of his hire and gets a special supply of calories. It is customary to bring hot meals and snacks to the harvest crew five times during the working day.

earlier evening meal. Now that most Americans work outside of the home, we all have similar eating habits; but our love of meat, potatoes, bread, and butter endures to this day.

Breakfast Cereal, the Father of Processed Foods

America became the perfect place to nurture the idea of 'quick and easy,' prepared foods. In an up-and-coming frontier country, and in the wake of the fast-moving industrial revolution, new concepts were admired and adopted.

In 1863, Dr. James Caleb Jackson created the first breakfast cereal, which he called *Granula*. It was marketed to replace old-fashioned porridge. In 1895, after quite a bit of experimentation, John Harvey Kellogg developed a cereal flake made of wheat, which he called *Granose*. By 1902, thirty different cereal companies had evolved, providing Americans with scores of cereals to choose from, each promising to cure their every ill.

So how did we end up with cold cereal, the almost universal American food of today? It started around 1920 when cooked cereals were first dried and toasted to make cold cereal, a thoroughly American innovation. Food manufacturers began to see the potential of ready-to-eat cereals for families who sent children off to school and parents off to work.

Shortly thereafter, companies developed and marketed canned soups for the same reasons. As easy as homemade soups are to make, they take time, which the modern, working family doesn't seem to have. So instead of preparing food fresh at home from local ingredients, the American diet shifted to foods based on mass production and distribution—and massive advertising. Radio, and then television, was developed for commercial use around the same time, powerful tools that helped convince Americans that they were too busy to cook. Then came the prepared-food conglomerates, a dominant force in shaping the modern American diet.

Fast-Foods for Today's Lifestyle

These food suppliers played right into the changing character of the American family life. Almost imperceptibly over the past few decades, our population has changed from the traditional married couple raising a family to an ever-increasing number of single parents, single young adults, and families where both parents work.

For couples raising families, economic growth added some additional important changes. Instead of children spending time just playing or doing homework, parents have felt the need to provide a wide spectrum of extra-curricular activities—gymnastics, music lessons, a variety of athletic activities, and much more—after school. Mothers, when not working, have become the taxi drivers, and while driving past attractive, brightly decorated, fast-food restaurants wafting the aroma of french fries, our homemade meals have been replaced by these fast-food giants and the prepared 'five-minute' microwave dishes.

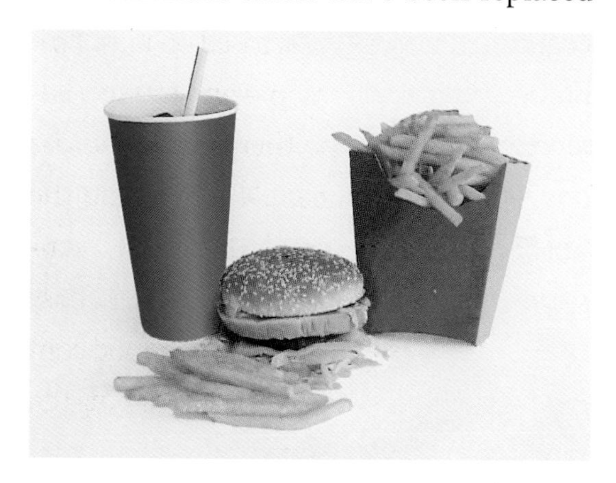

Children grow up fast and leave home earlier now, often without learning the basic skills they need like preparing and cooking food. Instead, they survive on processed, frozen, or canned foods and fast-foods from restaurants. If they learn cooking at all, they learn it through cookbooks, which are often written, ironically, by food manufacturers and processors.

Modern American Foods

Our taste preferences have shifted from the basic foods, as consumed by our ancestors, to the standardized flavors of processed foods, which are meaty, rich, and heavy and rooted in English origins. Seafood, vegetables, fruits, and other natural, wholesome foods, which are not easily processed for commercial purposes, are neglected; and worse, the processed foods are designed to please the average person and be affordable to everyone. As a result, we are overnourishing our bodies with a constant barrage of unhealthy, processed foods.

Winning Strategies

Humans develop their taste preferences very early in life. The brain of an infant can be compared to a new computer, and every new taste registers in the cell memory. If you give a child a wide assortment of different foods, he will grow up to like a variety of foods. On the other hand, if the child grows up eating a very limited selection of foods, especially mass-produced fast-foods, he will grow up with a taste for only those familiar foods. The smell, taste, and palate are all subjective, and they differ from individual to individual.

Years ago in Vienna, Austria, on the way to dinner one evening, I passed a street corner vendor with a cart roasting chestnuts. The aroma triggered the memory of a similar smell I had experienced as a child in Taiwan. My American companions were not impressed by the aroma. I could not resist, however, buying a package of those chestnuts. The memory has been with me ever since.

It is also interesting to note that at Nagasaki and Hiroshima, a few years after the atomic bomb explosions, the poor population had lower rates of cancers and radiation-related diseases than the affluent. During the war, most mechanical equipment was destroyed, and there was a shortage of refined foods like white rice. The poor people survived on unrefined rice and other similar foods. The simplicity of the poor people's diet was obviously better, health-wise, than that of the wealthy population who consumed the more rich and refined foods.

Conclusion

We have seen how Americans cultivated their love of meat, potatoes, bread, and butter as their preferred diet for the main meal. Vegetables, grains, and fruits never figured prominently in the American lifestyle. Today, when we can't have our favorite big meals, we turn to processed foods and fast-foods to tide us over to the next big meal, and this cycle affects our children. Many children are unaware that other options are available, or those options are ignored because they are reluctant to try something new and unfamiliar. But there is a way out.

It is logical to conclude that it takes a wide range of simple, natural, unrefined foods to stay healthy. For a nourishing diet, we need to know how to prepare a good variety of wholesome foods and to balance our ever-increasing reliance on processed and fast-foods.

We should train our children, from the beginning, about the healthy ways of eating and perhaps, in the process, retrain ourselves. This book provides the fundamentals with detailed, simple cooking techniques, which are easy to follow and incorporate into your daily routine.

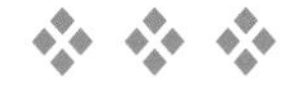

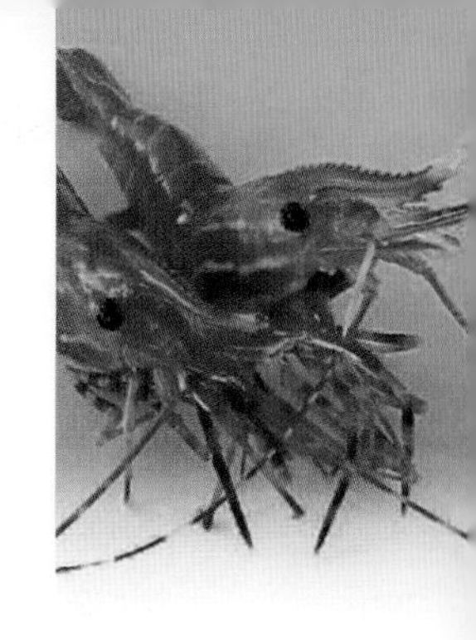

Chapter 2

Food Processing: A Lesson from the Shrimp

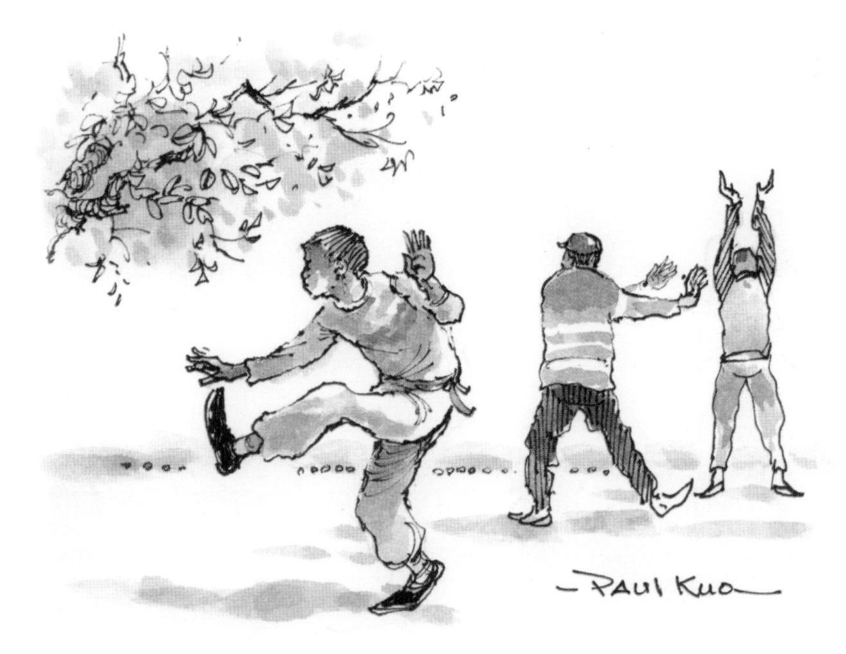

Even in this technological age, Tai Chi has become very popular among health conscious people around the world as a way to keep the mind and body strong and supple.

The Technological Revolution

Many of us have grown up in the middle of a huge scientific and technological revolution, especially during the last fifty years. This revolution has changed our lives completely, so now they are significantly different from our distant, or even our recent, ancestors. Most of these differences are wonderful, like medical advances, which save lives and minimize disease, and an abundance of consumer goods, including labor-saving devices, which give us plenty of leisure time to enjoy ourselves. We are accustomed to trusting technology; in fact, we bet our lives on it.

Some of our actions are astonishing. For example, we fly at 40,000 feet above the ground, near the speed of sound, inside a huge metal tube packed with hundreds of other humans, and we cruise at seventy-five miles an hour along a freeway. Millions of people live everyday with the belief, "In technology we trust," and don't even bother to say "Amen!" If we consider the worst-case scenario, we would all be a bit more pious. But at this point, we really have no choice but to trust technology.

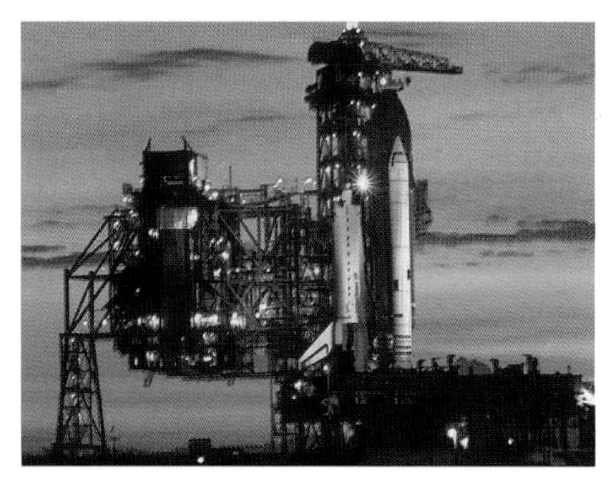

As a young engineer in the early 1970s, I participated with the Douglas Aircraft Company in the design of the DC-10 aircraft. We calculated the hardware that would be necessary to join together the DC-10's fuselage and wings, for the aircraft to make the takeoffs and landings expected during its designated life span. The bolts and structural pieces, which hold these critical parts together, are relatively minimal, and so, I always felt uneasy gambling people's lives on a few pieces of titanium. I used to fly only in Boeing 747s just because I didn't know the details of their design. Scientists reassure us that the airplanes are designed with plenty of margin for safety, and we count on that sort of reassurance everyday.

Danger of Depending on Technology

Because science and technology have developed to such a complex and refined state, we have no choice but to use and trust it—it's just too complicated for most of us to understand. This has created a potentially dangerous situation because in many aspects of our lives, we no longer trust our own judgment or think for ourselves. This tends to become part of our lifestyle. Instead, we trust so-called professionals or specialists to tell us what to do—or we have them do it for us. Without realizing it, as a population, we have become very institutionalized, and technology has institutionalized the most basic part of our life: the food we eat.

During this last half-century, we have become accustomed to eating a lot of processed foods. In spite of plentiful food supplies and a high quality of life, many of us suffer from a wide variety of unresolved medical problems, many of which

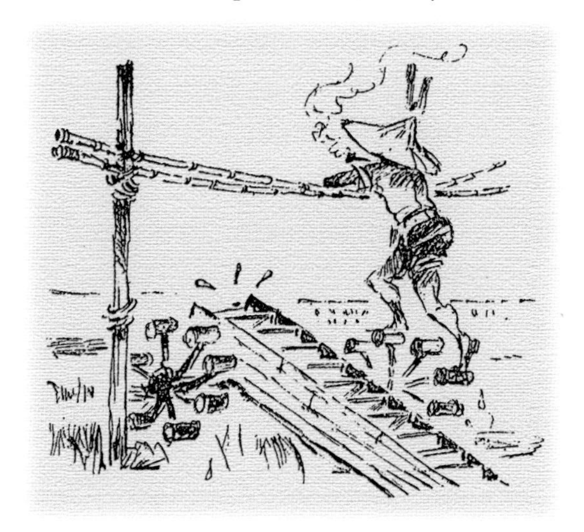

Waterwheel. This contented farmer eschews the gasoline pump and floods his paddy using a waterwheel completely made of wood. What was good enough for grandpa is good enough for him.

point to compromised immune systems. Medical experts agree that cancers, diabetes, allergies, and a host of other problems, including obesity, are related to immune system deficiencies.

For centuries, humans have eaten the food nature provides, until recently, when we started to apply modern technology and marketing to the food we eat. We adulterate our food to make it marketable, and in the process we have created new products that taste similar or better than natural food but are actually very different.

For example, french fries, onion rings, and chicken sandwich patties are reconstituted foods, that is, original, natural foods which have been altered to make them look and taste uniform. We can have french fries in Los Angeles in the springtime, or in New York in the summer, and they all taste and look alike. The processed chicken sandwich patties with added chemicals actually taste better to some people than natural chicken. We enjoy these foods and rarely question the potential, consequential health effects.

Differences between Natural and Processed Foods

So what are the differences between industrially processed foods and natural, unadulterated foods? Processed foods have a neutral taste and are cosmetically pleasing

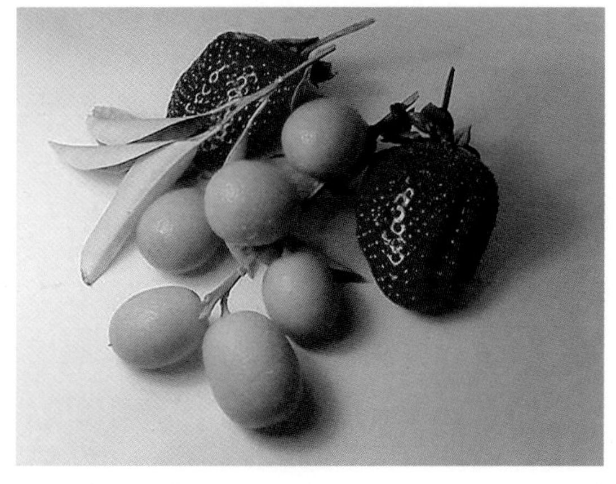

in color and texture; they are consistent and predictable, so they appeal to the masses. Natural foods generally have specific, characteristic tastes, smells, colors, and textures.

Processed, technologically-produced foods are designed to appeal to the broadest market and are easily acceptable to the mass palate. Unfamiliar, natural foods may necessitate an acquired taste. Nevertheless, they are whole foods with the balanced nutrients we need. In contrast, processed foods have one purpose: to make profits. Manufacturers make the food look and taste

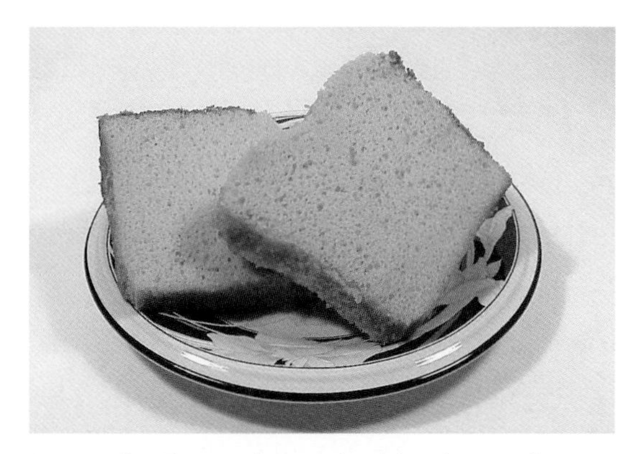

Green cake. The natural green color of this cake comes from juice squeezed out of coconut tree leaves, also adding to its flavor.

appealing, and then give it a brand name to make a profit from it.

Examples of Pharmaceutical Grade Foods with Elements Removed

Modern Table Salt

Salt has always been an important part of the human diet. Traditionally, when people lived far from the ocean, they paid premium prices for salt. It was even levied as a form of tax in some countries. We need salt to produce stomach acid so we can digest our food. It is also essential for proper brain function, nervous system health, and other important body functions. Even though some modern nutritionists warn us to stay away from salt, it is an essential part of our diet. Not many people realize that modern table salt is highly processed, totally different from the original salt that nature designed, the kind of salt our ancestors (from whom we get our genes) consumed.

When I arrived in America, I was overwhelmed by the quality of life. Even American salt was clean and orderly; the crystals poured out of the stylish and very civilized saltshaker like well-trained soldiers. In contrast, back home the salt was stored in a bowl with a tiny spoon. The crystals were usually gray, yellowish or pink, and of various sizes. The salt was always slightly damp; on a hot, humid day, you could sometimes see the water in the salt. Was this Taiwanese salt inferior, while Americans had the superior salt? Chemically, they are composed of mainly the same things. Our American salt is natural salt processed with modern technology and packaged nicely, ready-to-use with a well-known brand name. Salt in Taiwan is natural, unprocessed salt with no brand name. Taiwan has an abundant supply of salt since it is an island with plenty of seawater as a source.

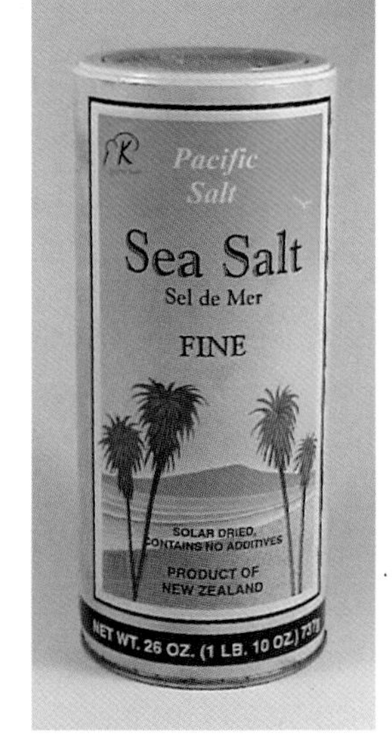

But this kind of salt is almost never used in America. The idea of commercializing this essence of human food is irresistible to American marketers. Salt is processed with high temperatures and other chemical processes, which include bleaching and the addition of a potentially harmful, aluminum-drying compound, a desiccant. The whole process removes valuable trace minerals such as magnesium, calcium, and potassium, all-important for our health. Magnesium is necessary for regulating our heart rhythm, and muscular and nervous systems. Having the right balance of minerals is essential for a healthy immune system.

Not all natural salts have the same chemical content because they are harvested in different localities. Traditional healers have always stressed that foods native to our locality are best for our health. But processed salt is a pure chemical, scientifically called sodium chloride. Scientists can simply react sodium (Na) with hydrochloric acid (HCl) to make salt (NaCl), although it is much cheaper to get salt from the ocean or from a salt dome. Because of refining and chemical additives, it is no longer natural salt; it has lost its original 'salt balance,' or, as the Chinese would say, its *yin-yang* balance. Prolonged consumption can deprive us of many important mineral elements in the natural salt, which can compromise our health, especially our immune system.

An interesting, historical example of refined salt causing problems was when the Hunza, a previously isolated people noted for their robust longevity, began to use refined salt. Their health deteriorated, and they began to live much shorter lives. It's all about marketing, so manufacturers can use a brand name to sell more salt. "When it rains, it pours," may be an accurate description of processed salt, but they don't mention that an aluminum desiccant is the chemical doing the trick. Interestingly, there are many kinds of less processed sea salts available in stores, especially in health food stores.

High-Tech, Refined Oil Vs. Natural Oil

We have the same problem with our modern cooking oils. Today, nutritionists blame fat intake for our overweight predicaments, but the problem is not that simple. Fat can come from animals or plants; in fact, most plants have some fat content, especially nuts and seeds.

In my youth, I observed oil-making first-hand because it was produced locally. The nuts or seeds were gently heated, then squeezed with a primitive machine to extract the oil. It takes a lot of nuts to get a bottle of oil. Cooking oil was one of the most expensive household items we had. The oil was filtered through a cloth and, after sitting in a bottle for

We get oil from the same materials as our ancestors, except we end up with a totally different and unwholesome product.

a few hours, the solid particles settled to the bottom. When there were enough nuts or seeds in our village, a small, local oil operation would produce the oil. The aroma penetrated for miles. For the children in our village, hungry most of the time, the smell drove us crazy! We stayed around to eat the pulp from the operation just like modern kids eat cookies. The pulp was still very oil-rich, and it tasted good to a hungry kid.

Today, oil is extracted with high-tech machines, which use a much higher-powered press, as well as non-edible chemical solvents, to make sure all of the oil is removed. The resulting solution is then distilled to remove the solvent. The solvent is recovered for reuse, but certain amounts are considered safe to remain in the oil for our consumption. Do they really know if these amounts that *remain* in the oil are actually safe?

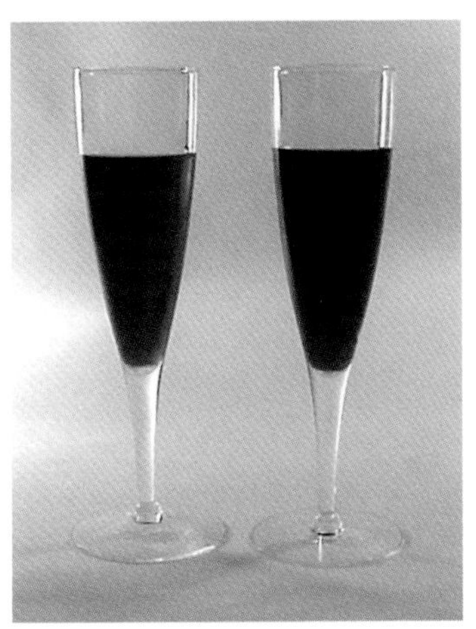

Sesame oil. High-tech (left) versus low-tech sesame oil; the differences are more than just the clarity of the oil; the taste is different.

The same technique is used to make all sorts of products from decaffeinated coffee to perfume. Many important elements naturally present in the nuts and seeds are removed and discarded because they are not cosmetically appealing. The oil is then further processed for clarity and aesthetic appearance. Like salt, oils and fats are essential to the daily diet, though modern experts say we should limit them severely. Many non-water-soluble nutrients require oil or fat for proper absorption. We get oil from the same materials as our ancestors, except we end up with a totally different and unwholesome product.

It's even worse when oils undergo hydrogenation to make margarine and similar products. A very toxic chemical, *nickel oxide*, is used as a catalyst for hydrogenation. After complex manipulation, and the addition of toxic chemicals, we end up with hydrogenated oil. The solid oil is then bleached and color is added for aesthetics. This solid cooking oil is easier to package than liquid oil, easier to use, and has a longer shelf life. The hydrogenation rearranges the chemicals in the oils, but our bodies can't recognize the structure of the fatty-acid chains, so we end up with health problems, including obesity.

This hydrogenated oil is a common ingredient in many commercial and processed foods. Hydrogenated fats like margarine may be one of the most harmful foods available today. Health experts agree that hydrogenated fats may contribute to heart and circulatory ailments.

Nevertheless, fat is still a major issue among nutritionists who all say to avoid 'bad' fat (animal fat) and consume 'good' fat (vegetable oil). As previously indicated, technologically produced oils are not as healthy as we would like. The most recent research indicates that the short-chain fatty acids like those in butter and cream, nuts and seeds, and other animal fats are necessary for our diet and especially essential for growing children.

In the early days when the economy was simple and primitive in Taiwan, we could not just go to the market and buy everything we needed ready-made. For cooking, my mother used to buy a piece of pork belly, all white and fat. She cut it into small pieces and rendered the fat slowly over low heat, salted lightly, and then strained it into a jar. If we slaughtered a fat chicken, duck, or goose, the fat portion at the bottom of the fowl was always made into cooking fat. The solids, left over after rendering, were cooked with vegetables; it tasted like bacon. When the rendered fat cooled down, it became semi-solid; a substance you know as lard.

In early Taiwan, most of the population consumed such animal fat because vegetable oils were expensive; yet we rarely saw anyone overweight or suffering health problems associated with eating animal fat. Even lard or other animal fats were expensive, and the amount used in cooking was appropriate. Nobody can abuse foods that are in short supply! However, the poorest people, who could not afford even lard to cook their foods, developed vitamin deficiency diseases including night blindness and gum disease.

Glory Days of MSG

The Japanese developed MSG, or *monosodium glutamate*, in the early twentieth century. It's a naturally occurring salt of glutamic acid, called glutamate, extracted from seaweed or sugar beets. Glutamate is found in protein-rich foods such as aged cheeses, meat, and fish. The Japanese call the savory, meat-like flavor of MSG '*Ajinomoto*,' literally, 'the essence of taste.' There is no English word for this taste. We can describe it as 'brothy,' or 'meaty,' or 'savory,' but an easier way to experience how it tastes is to sprinkle your tongue with parmesan cheese. The

Japanese regard this flavor as the fifth basic flavor, in addition to sweet, sour, bitter, and salty.

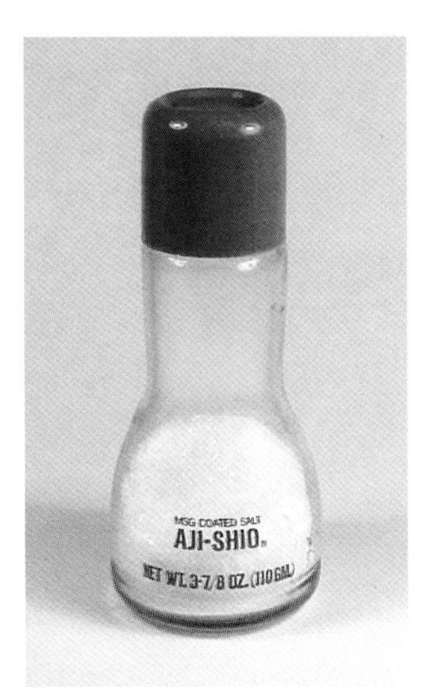

Recently, researchers identified the exact protein molecule on our taste buds that reacts to the glutamine flavor, which is the stimulus that helps us distinguish and seek out high protein food. The company that invented the method of producing MSG is still in business today: Ajinomoto Food Company. In fact, the Taiwanese still call MSG "Ajinomoto." It was very expensive prior to the 1960s and, as I recall, only the wealthy could afford it.

My father was a policeman in Japanese-occupied Taiwan. It was the custom for merchants to give gifts to policemen during holidays like New Year's. We used to receive our annual supply of MSG on New Year's Day. When we visited our grandparents in their very remote village, the gift of a small can of Ajinomoto made them very happy, and they proudly showed it to their neighbors and friends. When my mother cooked, I remember her dabbing tiny portions of it into certain, special dishes.

In the 1960s, new techniques were developed to produce MSG, and it became very inexpensive. Today, MSG costs about the same as table salt. In the old days, it was packaged in very small bottles, less than one ounce; but now, we buy it by the pound. Because it enhances flavors so well, and so cheaply, food processors overuse and abuse it.

One day, I watched a fast-food cook liberally sprinkle MSG from a big container all over a batch of french fries, and I was shocked. He must have used 100 times the amount my mother used when I was a child. But today, the average Taiwanese consumes about 2.4 pounds of MSG a year, the highest per capita consumption. However, that may include the MSG in exported, processed foods. Ironically, it was never popular in Mainland China due, no doubt, to their depressed economy during most of the past century. In America, however, MSG is identified with Chinese restaurants.

MSG has a bad reputation for causing allergic reactions and making some people sick, but when used properly, there is nothing wrong with MSG. According to a recent FDA report, MSG has no adverse health effects when used appropriately. For example, in the year 2000, a study conducted at the Scripps Research Institute in La Jolla, California showed that large doses of MSG were no more likely to cause a reaction in asthmatics than a placebo.

The World Health Organization, the Food and Drug Administration, and the Scientific Committee for Food of the European Commission have all concluded that human studies have failed to confirm the existence of 'the Chinese restaurant syndrome.' MSG is on the World Health Organization's list of 'safest foods,' along with vinegar and salt. The problem is that we abuse it. Ajinomoto is a safe flavoring, and I still use it on most dishes.

Certain foods contain a lot of glutamate naturally, which is one reason these foods taste so good. A pizza with tomato sauce and parmesan cheese tastes good because it is rich in glutamate. There are other ways to achieve this natural MSG flavor. For example, bonito is a type of fish most people will not eat. The Japanese cook this fish until all odors disappear, and then dry it. The processed, dried bonito looks and feels as hard as wood. Once prepared, it is shaved with a sharp blade and used to season vegetables, or it can be powdered and added to soup. It adds that same 'savory' taste as MSG, and it's all natural and high in protein. This bonito fish stock, processed with salt and other ingredients, then made into granules, is a very popular form of seasoning for cooking as well as making soup.

Most fine restaurants claim not to use MSG, but their food still has that 'savory' taste because they make their stock with bones.

Food or Medicine?

We have the same problem with sugar. The underlying problem with processing food is that we insist on refining foods to an artificial standard of purity. We process food like we produce medicines. The result is that basic foods like salt and sugar are more like medicine than food because they are produced as nearly pure chemicals. They lack the natural balancing elements we need for good health.

It seems that our troubles with cocaine stem from the same problem. This horrible substance has caused untold suffering. For generations, the Peruvians have been chewing coca leaves as an important food to help them function in their high altitude, bad weather, and harsh living conditions. They don't have ill effects from chewing the leaves. But like sugar and salt, and other processed foods, cocaine is extracted from the coca leaves with solvent and then distilled for purity and high potency. The resulting purified cocaine is now a chemical, not a food. Our bodies are genetically programmed to consume foods as nature provided, unadulterated and unconcentrated. Food and technology just don't always mix for good health.

Healthy Diets, an Oxymoron

The first dieting book was written in 1836, probably for the rich population who had plenty to eat and lived high. Today, there are about 15,400 diet books on the market, a grand cacophony of diet methods, which, when combined with all the diet foods and supplements, make for a multi-billion dollar industry. The U.S. government has announced that none of these fad diets are really effective, and that the only way to lose weight is to control one's caloric intake. The results of this dieting craze have been disappointing, and we are still struggling with obesity and related health problems. As Americans, why do we have such a hard time with our nutrition? We will probably never see a truly effective, short-term diet solution.

A Lesson from the Shrimp

This massive effort to lose weight reminds me of an interesting lesson I learned some years ago. In the early 1960s, as part of the national economic development program, Taiwan began a research project to produce shrimp, a popular delicacy worldwide. It's hard to harvest shrimp predictably from the ocean, so they decided to

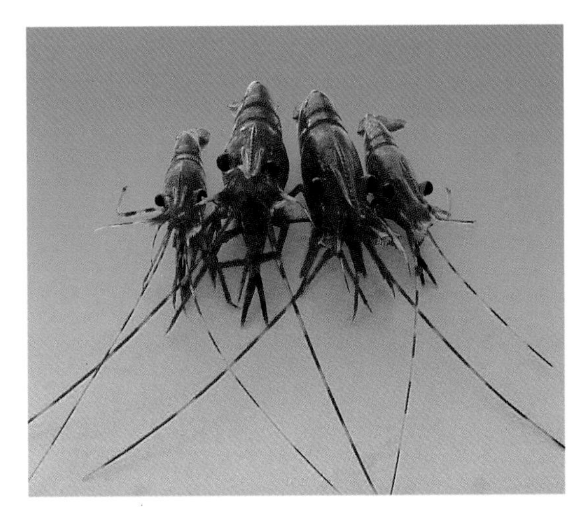

If overfed, they overeat and die.
If underfed or fed too late, the baby shrimp eat their own tails, and then die.

grow it. The price of quality shrimp was very good at the time, so a successful program to produce shrimp for the market could be an economic bonanza and a good source of U.S. dollars for Taiwan. As with any animal farming, the baby shrimp needed to be produced in large quantities.

There was very little scientific information available at that time to help solve the problem of massive shrimp egg production. Without scientific theory, Taiwanese scientists tried different ways of making it happen until, one day, a female shrimp's eye was accidentally snapped off. To the astonishment of the scientists, after a few days, this shrimp started to produce a lot of eggs. So they decided to remove the other eye, and the shrimp produced even more eggs. This accidental discovery made the shrimp aquaculture program successful, and we have enjoyed a good supply of tiger shrimp ever since.

When the shrimp first hatch, they are almost microscopic in size. You really need a keen pair of eyes to see them. They need constant, skillful care, twenty-four hours a day. The tiny shrimp have to be fed specially prepared food, exactly on time, and in the proper amounts. If overfed, they overeat and die. If underfed or fed too late, the baby shrimp eat their own tails, and then die.

When I first heard this story from a relative, who made his fortune as one of the first pioneers in shrimp aquaculture, it made me think about our human behavior. If a shrimp had a logical mind, it would never eat itself for quick satisfaction only to die a few minutes later. Unfortunately, shrimp don't have much common sense. They have a shrimp mentality, and sometimes I wonder if we humans suffer from the same outlook.

What do I mean by a shrimp mentality? I mean our need for instant gratification, no matter what the price we may pay later on. Or more simply, it means, "Do it now, worry about it later." For example, we buy expensive items with 'no down payment,' 'no payment until June,' and we use our credit cards to do it, ignoring the fact that we have to pay later with a very high interest rate. But we prefer to enjoy the gratification now and not worry about what comes later. Today, we are obsessed with dieting, and our approach to solving weight problems is much like the shrimp eating themselves to satisfy their hunger.

Instant Weight Loss

Fat tissue is part of everyone's body mass. It is not a dumbbell that we can just drop and walk away from. The extra weight we don't like is part of nature's way of conserving energy in case of need. This extra weight is part of our body, so if we want to get rid of it, we need to do it with consideration for our overall well-being instead of just taking a pill or using oversimplified, abusive methods, which produce extreme weight loss in a short time. Any quick, short-term weight loss abuses the body system, not to mention the possible long-term consequences, damage to our health

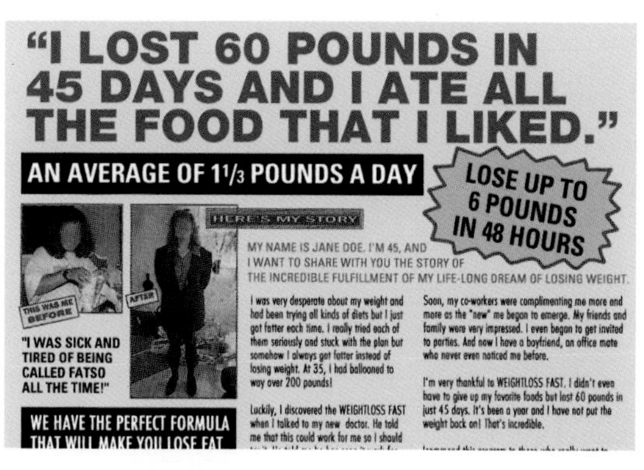

through excessive and quick aging, muscle loss, electrolyte imbalances, and similar problems. People who lose ten pounds in one week are very happy, but they don't care that they may have aged six months in the process. Common sense tells us that any method of weight loss needs to be effective over time, and permanent, and the only way to accomplish this goal is to change our lives sensibly so we continue to enjoy good health as we do it.

Simple Minded

In our scientific world, we all know that nature provides foods with complex, well-balanced substances for our health. Yet we insist on refining the foods we eat into pure, simple chemicals. Take calcium for example, an element in the periodic table. It is very poisonous to humans in its pure state. In foods, as well as in our bodies, it exists as calcium compounds in various forms. But we are advised to take calcium pills made up of calcium carbonate or seashells (found in anti-acids), or to drink milk.

Milk is rich in calcium, but milk may have undesirable side effects. Taking a pill and drinking milk may not supply all the varieties of calcium compounds and other mineral compounds we need. Foods provided by nature contain a wide variety of balanced mineral compounds in a form our bodies can assimilate. Heavy dark-green vegetables are very rich in calcium and other mineral compounds. The wise approach is to eat a variety of foods, to make soup stock with animal bones, and to eat seafood and vegetables.

Trying to eat a fat-free diet is a similar example. As I mentioned previously, right after WWII, there was a food shortage in Taiwan. I observed, firsthand, that the poor people did not get sufficient fat in their diet and suffered many health problems such as dull skin, bloated stomachs, and a lack of muscle elasticity.

Vitamins A, D, and E occur naturally in various compounds, and they are not water-soluble; these vitamins need fat or oil for proper absorption. Vitamins B and C are water-soluble and also consist of many different compounds. Vitamin C from orange juice can be a different variety of the vitamin C from spinach, and our body needs all varieties of vitamins.

Too Lazy to Do It Right

We all know that healthy food and exercise are the price we must pay for good health. The equation for losing weight is very simple: eat balanced foods, eat smaller portions, and cut down on fast-foods and sweets while eating less to control weight.

With this approach and exercise, we can maintain good health easily—and we lose weight. Remember, while losing weight, our body still needs proper nutrients to function. But many of us try to get around it with drastic diet regimens or diet pills. Our recent disaster with Fen-Phen is a good example of what our shrimp mentality is doing to our health. To put it simply, we need to know how to prepare natural, fresh, balanced meals, which allow us to manipulate our weight (up or down) while staying healthy and enjoying one of the best parts of being alive—a delicious meal.

Consequence of Affordable Fast-Foods

As the world's economy becomes more and more global, the American style of fast-food has proliferated throughout the world. This, however, is something of a Trojan horse. You can see this most dramatically among populations that, until very recently, had eaten traditional, natural foods and then turned to American processed fast-food. For example, when American fast-food started to gain popularity in China, in less than ten years, we saw the children of the affluent, who could afford the American fast-foods, become overweight. Instead of avoiding American fast-food and returning to their traditional foods, weight management clinics for children sprung up in many of the major cities. What a shrimp mentality!

Similarly, on Tonga in Polynesia, the King holds the *Guinness World Book of Records* for being the heaviest monarch in the world. This island has a population of 100,000, and the majority of the population is so overweight that diabetes is a universal problem. The King admitted that the entire island loves American food, especially hamburgers and hot dogs.

Recognizing the health risks to the population, the government began offering money to reward people who lost weight. The more pounds they lost, the more money they received. Many of the islanders went back to their traditional diets and started losing weight. The King, however, confessed that he had a very hard time giving up American fast-food, and he's still the heaviest monarch in the world.

Vulnerable Population

This problem on Tonga illustrates a general trend that I have noticed; most traditional populations seem to maintain a healthy weight until they discover American junk food. Evidence confirms that this is also true with American populations. For example, most Native Americans were traditionally lean and strong until incarceration on reservations eliminated their natural food sources and made them rely on American foods. African-Americans suffered through several generations of turmoil and discontinuity of their traditional cooking, which ultimately resulted in a diet heavily adapted from modern processed foods or fast-foods.

Many of these Americans have lost their link with traditional healthy cooking and eating. As a result, these groups of Americans, according to doctors from the Centers for Disease Control and Prevention, have the highest rates of Type 2 diabetes in the world. Obese Americans often eat a great deal of fast-food, especially when both parents work, or a single mother has to work many hours to support her family.

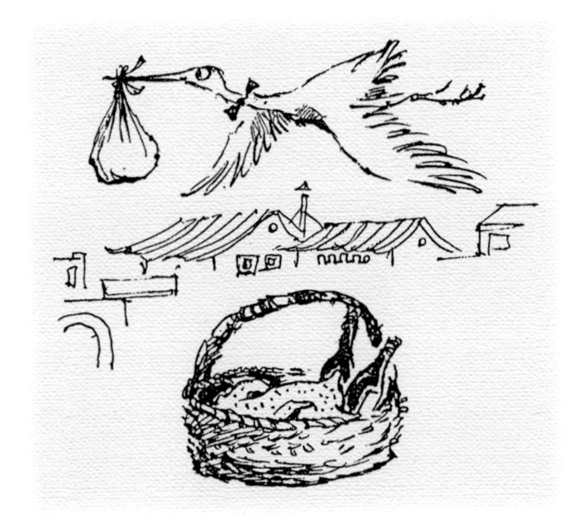

Supplementary diet. Immediately on the birth of a child, the maternal grandparents send the new mother a gift; bottles of rice wine and a rooster cooked with sesame oil. The old custom is probably predicated on just plain common sense.

In Hawaii, an American-Japanese doctor convinced his overweight patients suffering from diabetes to go back to their traditional diet based on native, starchy foods. Most of them lost the weight and overcame their diabetic symptoms. It's depressing to think that the science and technology in which we have placed our trust has betrayed us. Companies have mishandled science and technology for their business purposes, and most of us have bought right into it. We demand foods that are quick, refined, and cosmetically pleasing. And there you have a shrimp mentality!

Interesting Old Custom

Even though my mother never attended school, lived through both the Japanese and Chinese occupations in Taiwan, and has lived in the United States for the last twenty years, she knows the difference between foods that promote health and foods that do not. She always complains that the refined foods we eat do not taste natural and seem unhealthy.

There is an old Taiwanese belief that eating chicken cooked with sesame oil, rice wine, and ginger will help a nursing mother provide plenty of rich, healthy milk for her baby. Years ago, when my mother-in-law learned we were expecting our first baby, she hatched a couple of batches of chicks. She timed the maturing of the chickens with the due date of the baby. As soon as the child arrived, all twenty chickens were delivered in cages to Taipei from her remote village. My mother killed one every other day.

It only took a few days for my wife to get sick of eating sesame chicken, day in and day out, so I was the one enjoying sesame chicken for a month. But my wife ate some, and she really did have plenty of milk for our baby, even though she only weighed a hundred pounds.

A few years ago, when my daughter-in-law Charlotte was expecting her first child, my mother returned from Taiwan with a large bottle of sesame oil made in the traditional way by people she knew in the village. The oil was thick, heavy, and cloudy with a natural sesame smell. It looked primitive, but my mother insisted that it was healthy food for the mother and child.

The sesame oil we buy from the stores in America is clear and sanitized, with very little sesame odor. It's a shame that the elders of the previous generations are passing away, and we have not learned from them to cook with unrefined, unprocessed foods. It was impossible to convince an all-American girl like Charlotte to eat chicken cooked with the Taiwanese oil.

Today, many ethnic stores still carry basic, homegrown, unprocessed foods. Many of our friends from India frequently visit Indian stores to purchase spices like curry. These unprocessed, natural foods have no brand names and they come primitively packaged. Often these ethnic stores are the only places to buy natural foods. Even in the health food stores, real unrefined oils are rare. If you grow up eating unrefined, natural food, you sense that there is something wrong with the processed foods in fancy packages.

In contrast, young people growing up today are accustomed to new products with fancy packages, and they won't touch unprocessed foods, which seem unsanitary, primitive, and unappetizing. Even so, I think we should do our best to find natural, unrefined products, and cook our everyday meals with them. Over time, this 'natural' diet can help restore our ideal health.

Chapter 3

Old Wisdom

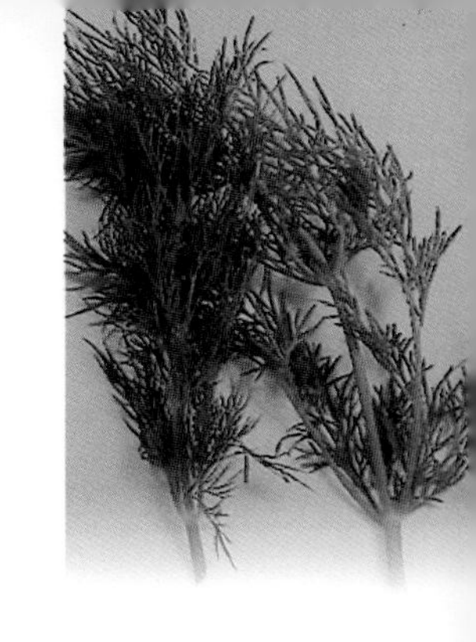

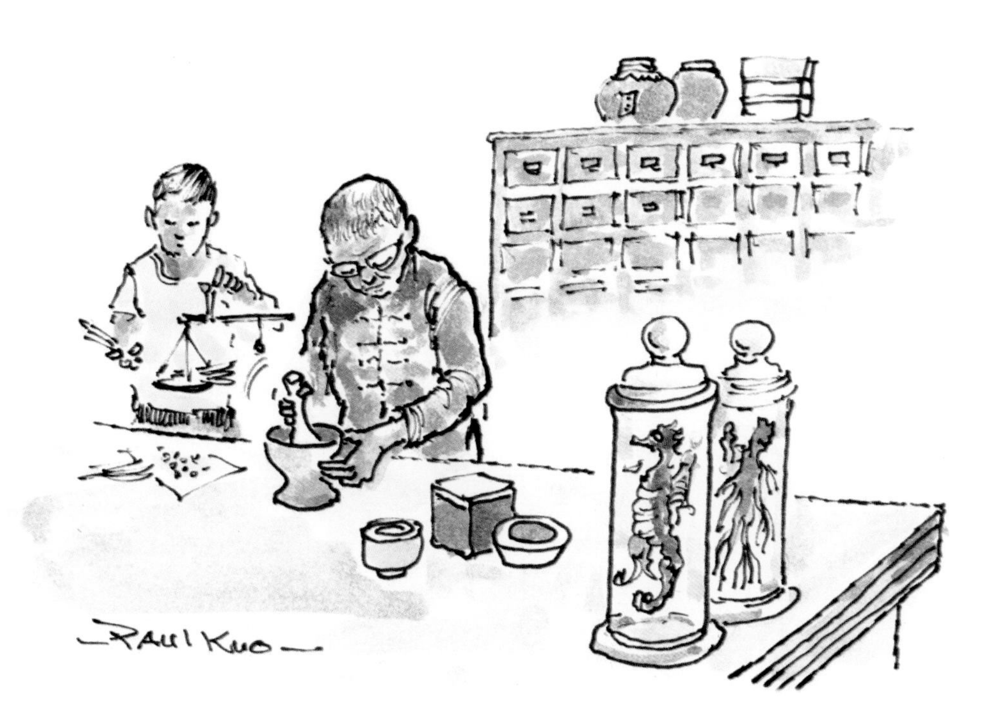

When you think about it, America is a *very* new nation. Even our oldest settlements are only a few hundred years old. Many other cultures have thrived much longer, over thousands of years. Most of our ancestors arrived here only a few generations ago; and when they arrived, most of them entered a new culture and landed right in the middle of an industrial or technological revolution. Suddenly, they were in the midst of a lifestyle that had never existed on earth before.

New Knowledge and Old Wisdom

Much of this new lifestyle is positive—a medical technology that has doubled our life span; affordable, accessible travel, which has allowed a whole population to move about economically and easily; and technology that has given us abundant, affordable luxuries of all kinds.

After just a few generations in this new culture, however, many of us have lost the roots of our cultural traditions. We may forget that there are two parts of human knowledge: the new things we learn ourselves from daily experiences and the old wisdom passed down from generation to generation.

In our fast-paced modern life, we often forget and neglect the traditional wisdom our ancestors accumulated over thousands of years. Much of this wisdom was the product of experience and observation. It's easy to understand why we turn our backs on the old wisdom: it seems all our needs are met in this modern lifestyle, so who needs the old ways? I think we all do, and many people today are beginning to feel the same.

The great American humorist Mark Twain once noted that when he was fourteen, he was sure his father was an idiot but by the time he was twenty-one, he was astonished at how much the old man had learned. And I agree. I think we would marvel at the wisdom of our ancestors if only we would stop and listen. We all know that with the old wisdom came certain prejudices and superstitions. We moderns tend to reject these and, unfortunately, we throw the baby out with the bath water; that is, we don't stop to consider whether some of the old ways were wise and worth adopting.

Today, there are numerous conditions that medical science just can't seem to cure. Obesity is one of them. For all our technological advances, Americans still struggle with weight control. We must eat every day; there's no way around it. But obesity is recognized as one of the most prevalent health problems today, and modern science hasn't offered a viable solution to our overweight dilemma—but traditional wisdom has some answers. I think it's smart to pay attention to what traditional wisdom has to say about nutrition. Why? Because we have inherited body systems that are programmed to perform well on what our ancestors ate.

Medicinal Value of Foods

Over the centuries, every culture developed a body of medical knowledge to ease pain, suffering, and to heal people. This developed partially from our survival instinct—shared with the animal world—and partly from our gift of human compassion. But with the absence of modern medical knowledge, the healing arts were very limited. Physicians had few options other than herbal medicines and spiritual practices to

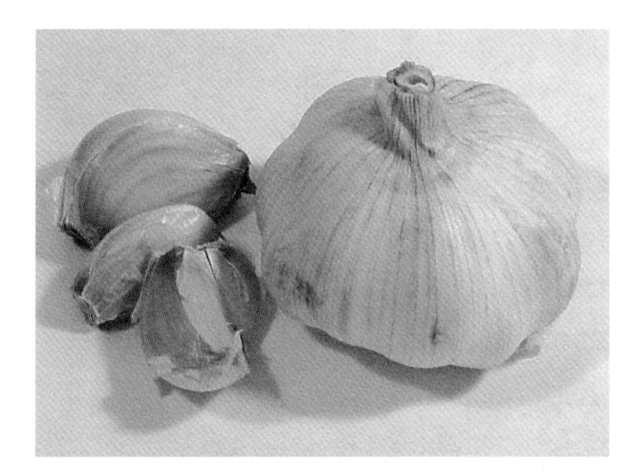

heal their patients, but they advised their patients about the foods and drinks they should consume. Therefore, eating healthy food was much more important to people of earlier times than it is today.

Over the millennia, our predecessors developed an abstract dietary theory about the physiology of digestion, the nutritive as well as medicinal properties of foodstuffs, and the nature of a healthy meal. This old wisdom passed from generation to generation was modified along the way and is still faithfully practiced by most ethnic cultures, except for us modern thinkers, all over the world. Today, we use our newly acquired knowledge about foods based on calories, vitamins, fiber content, and fat grams. The old dietary wisdom of the past is ignored almost entirely and considered old-fashioned. Food is fuel and pleasure, that's all.

If you eat a meal with someone from a traditional culture such as an Asian culture, it's hard to avoid a discussion about the health and medicinal properties of the dishes on the table, such as the medicinal benefits of the individual ingredients: mushrooms, shark fin, internal organs, and the way the dishes were prepared for maintaining a proper equilibrium of '*chi*' and *yin/yang* balance. Perhaps these conversations are mostly an exchange of polite pleasantries, but we still wonder, is there any validity to this kind of thinking? If we simply ignore it, perhaps we are merely disrespectful, but are we missing a valuable lesson?

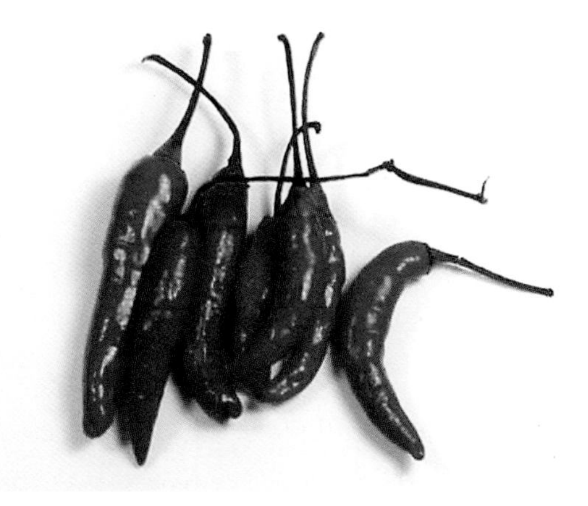

Chinese Medical Wisdom: Yin and Yang in Balance

It may be difficult at first to understand the old traditions and see their relevance to our lives today. But if we can be a little open-minded, we may begin to see that our ancestors' wisdom can be of practical use to us today. Let's take a look at traditional Chinese medicine as an example. Chinese history is relatively easy to track because their traditional culture spans five thousand years of written history, preserved because the Chinese have had the printing press for centuries. This made it easy to pass along knowledge from one generation to the next.

Unfortunately, the accumulated years of such information resulted in a complex, abstract, and ambiguous system, which

"A Chinese doctor diagnoses a patient by finding the imbalances... by feeling the intensity, speed, and rhythm of the pulse."

includes telling fortunes, predicting natural and human disasters, and a complicated system of medical theories.

Although Chinese medicine is complex, it has proven effective through generations for over thousands of years. The basic concept of Chinese medicine is founded on the idea that health results from physical and mental 'balance' within a person's body and also within the environment.

Traditional Chinese medicine strives to regain and maintain this same balance and harmony. The terms 'yin' and 'yang' describe such a balance, and these concepts are used to describe the factors that must be kept in balance; that is, the goal is to avoid an excess of either. A value of 'yin' or 'yang' is ascribed to various conditions, foods, herbs, etc.

In nature, we are surrounded by opposite pairs: male and female, dark and light, warm and cold, night and day, sun and moon, and so on. These opposites are not absolute but, instead, are understood in relation to each other. When we are healthy, yin and yang exist in balance. If they slip out of balance, the result is disease. So the logical conclusion must be this: to regain your health, you need to regain your balance.

A Chinese doctor diagnoses a patient by finding the imbalances. He does this by feeling the intensity, speed, and rhythm of the pulse. He also examines the coating and condition of the tongue, facial complexion, and other external factors. Taking the patient's condition into consideration, the doctor makes a final diagnosis and prescribes treatments to balance the body.

The Chinese pharmacopoeia was established through trial and error over thousands of years based on these very theories. The medicines are derived from botanical, animal, and mineral sources, and include the medicinal properties of food. The adage "Food is medicine" has always been a part of the Chinese culture, which teaches

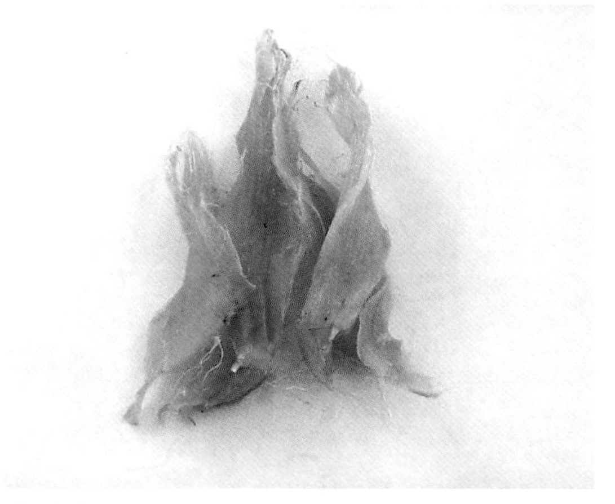

Shark fin. In China, shark fin is not only a delicacy but it's also believed to contain anti-cancer and anti-tumor elements, which medical research has just recently verified.

that foods can cure illness or cause illness. One's daily diet needs to have a balance of yin and yang, and if we can master the application of this theory in practice, we can enjoy optimal health. In traditional Chinese medicine, this can get pretty complex, and most of us can become lost trying to apply it to our everyday lives. We can simplify the concept, however, so that we can easily apply it to our lives.

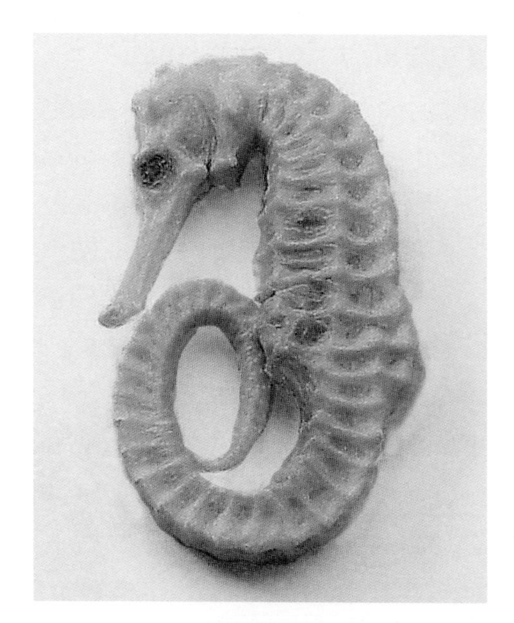

Boo Yao wine. Try a couple sake cups of this Chinese favorite wine (seahorse and herbs steeped in rice wine) before bedtime; it revitalizes and soothes the body, and it's an aphrodisiac as well.

Similar Concepts from the West

The notion of a balanced human constitution occurs throughout the world and not just in Chinese medicine. Many cultures taught that the human body is a microcosm of the universe and is composed of, and influenced by, the same elements present throughout the natural world. The Chinese identified five elements: water, fire, wood, metal, and earth. If you try to read about all of this in detail, the concepts may seem rather fuzzy and difficult to understand unless you spend enough time learning what the terms really mean.

Similar concepts, however, have influenced European and British medical philosophy. For example, in ancient Greece, Hippocrates and Galen taught the 'Doctrine of the Four Humors,' which became the most powerful concept in medieval, medical thinking. The Tudors believed that everything was made up of four elements: earth, air, fire, and water (which resembles the Chinese five elements). The earth was considered dry, water was moist, fire was hot, and air was cold. Foods were divided by their qualities into different degrees of hot and cold, similar to the Chinese yin and yang. It's easy to see how these concepts relate to Chinese philosophy. The Tudors also considered the types of foods one's ancestors were accustomed to eating. Certain nationalities could eat things that were bad for others. Thus, beer was a good drink for the Dutch, but a bad one for Englishmen since the English national drink was ale, which was brewed differently from beer.

Too Scientific for Our Health

As you can see, nutritional theory in different parts of the world during ancient times was astonishingly similar. In contrast, today we only consider foods based on certain scientifically identified, nutritional values: proteins, calories, carbohydrates, vitamins, and so on. We assume that as long as the nutrients are there, we can eat any food, and our bodies will take care of the digestion and absorption.

As mentioned before, we treat our bodies as if they are machines. Just as feeding high-octane gasoline into an engine will make it run, putting nutrients into our bodies will make us well. For instance, we are told that drinking lots of orange juice will give us an ample supply of vitamin C, which will help us avoid colds and maintain our general health. Based on the old wisdom, orange juice is classified as having cold and damp energy; too much could make people sick. It's true for me—I can only take so much orange juice.

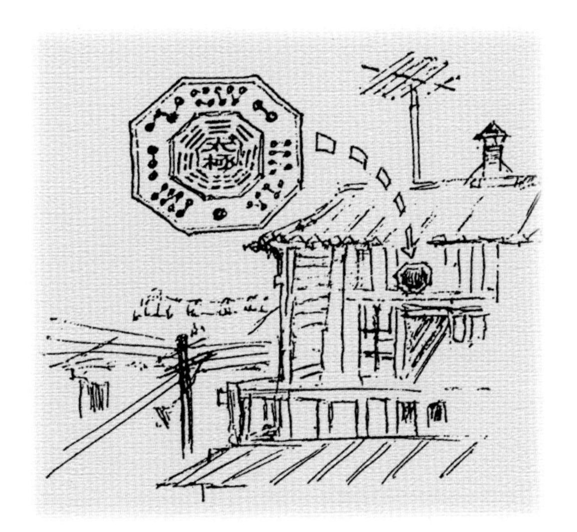

Good luck sign. This curious good luck sign is often placed on houses to ward off ill fortune caused by larger structures being erected on the opposite side of the street. Often a simple pocket mirror strategically placed will do the trick.

Similarly, in western thought, everybody thinks that eating sweet foods, which contain high calories, will make us gain weight. In contrast, the Chinese concept teaches that sweet foods promote digestive function and are, therefore, beneficial to people with a weak digestive system.

Things are different today, of course, because instead of unrefined sweets, we are talking about refined, pure sugar, which is many times sweeter and not as wholesome as natural sweets. Still, totally abstaining from sweets is probably an unnecessary sacrifice.

Traditional nutrition also considers the action of foods. For example, mature ginger is pungent and hot and has the property of outward movement. At the onset of a cold, when we feel weak, a cup of strong, warm, fresh ginger soup with some honey warms our body and the outward energy of the ginger makes us perspire, increasing blood circulation and we feel better, which also improves our immune system's ability to fight the cold. Warm ginger soup or ginger candy is commonly used in winter to

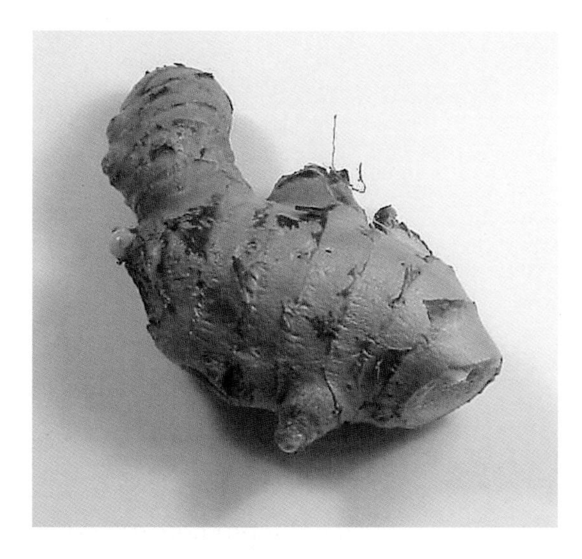

warm the body. On hot summer days or after vigorous exercise on a hot day, most of us want to drink ice-cold beer or a cold soft drink. Old wisdom tells us to eat watermelon (or any melon), sugarcane juice with some herbs added, or lemonade with a little honey to remove the heat energy from within the body. As you can see, the old wisdom taught, "You are what you eat," and bore in mind that foods have medicinal properties.

Body Warmer Tradition

As a child growing up in Taiwan, I remember the annual ritual at the year's end. During the year, my mother raised a flock of ducklings—a special variety of duck that was considered to have heat energy. The mature male had a red face, and he was incredibly strong and very sexually active.

On the shortest day of the year, about a week before Christmas, which signaled the coming of winter, my mother cooked one of the strongest male ducks with very hot, dry, yang ingredients. She mashed mature ginger roots and strained the juice. She cut the duck into small pieces, no more than a couple of inches each, and slow-cooked it with ginger juice, rice wine, and some hot herbs like cinnamon twigs. She added no water or regular wine since these were recognized for cold energy or yin properties.

At about midnight, my mother woke all eight of us children and gave us a couple of pieces of the meat with broth. The strong, pungent, hot, spicy taste warmed our bodies and helped us resist winter cold and dampness. It helped protect our bodies throughout the entire winter. Similarly, science has recently found that chicken soup does actually alleviate cold symptoms, if not help cure a cold.

Best of Both Worlds

These philosophies of old wisdom evolved from very early times with foods prescribed as medicines. Traditional medicine evaluated foods by how they affected our body systems and not just on their nutritional content. Today, we have almost lost touch with this kind of approach and focus instead just on the nutritional content of foods. While we are not likely to adopt many of the old superstitions interwoven into folk tradition, it's still a good idea to look at the traditional view, and see how it might benefit us. In fact, it's really easy to use the best of both worlds.

Modern recipes emphasize foods that look good and taste good. Traditional cooking looks at more than just the taste and appearance; instead, it considers balancing our foods for ideal health. It is based more on principles than on specific ingredients.

In this book, we endeavor to describe these principles, the basic and easy rules of balancing yin and yang. You don't need complicated recipes to eat this way, just a few simple principles and techniques. We have provided these techniques, and some easy-to-follow instructions for how to use these traditional ways of cooking in our fast, modern lifestyle. The result? Better health for you and your family.

PART TWO

Food for Thought: Modern Foods

As omnivores, our bodies are conditioned to digest a wide variety of foods. Until relatively recent times, nature provided the foods we ate. But in just a few decades, new technologies and scientific concepts applied to our foods have taken them well beyond what nature provides. Without our being totally aware of it, the constitution of the foods we typically eat has drastically changed. While our digestive and immune systems have evolved over eons, adapting over time, there are clear indications that our body systems are not adapting well to the relatively sudden changes in our diet. So despite these scientific advances, we encounter new health problems and cannot uncover their cause.

The experts all tell us that, next to genetics, diet has a substantial impact on health, but not all agree on what a healthy diet might be. Small wonder there is an unending parade of diet books populating the best-seller lists! Everyone is searching for 'the truth,' but where does it lie? It makes good sense for us to take a closer look at the major changes made to our foods and diets in recent years, concentrating on raw vegetable salads and the impact of technology on meat production and food processing.

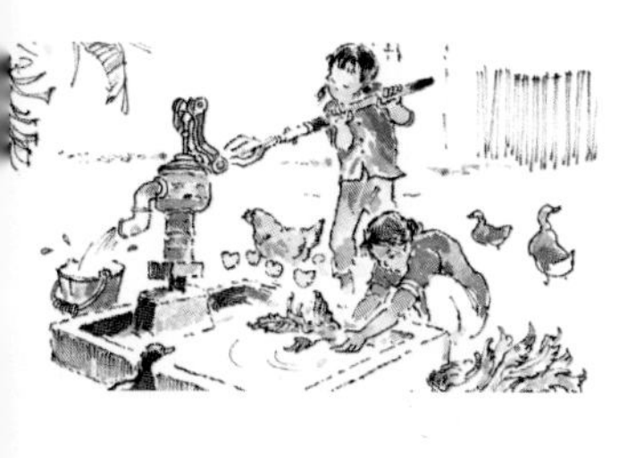

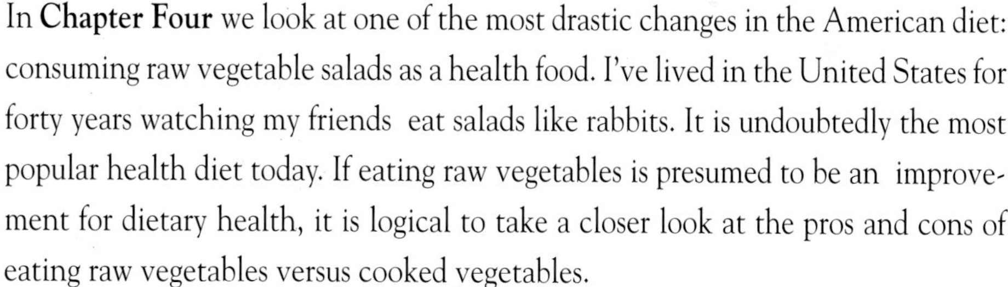

In **Chapter Four** we look at one of the most drastic changes in the American diet: consuming raw vegetable salads as a health food. I've lived in the United States for forty years watching my friends eat salads like rabbits. It is undoubtedly the most popular health diet today. If eating raw vegetables is presumed to be an improvement for dietary health, it is logical to take a closer look at the pros and cons of eating raw vegetables versus cooked vegetables.

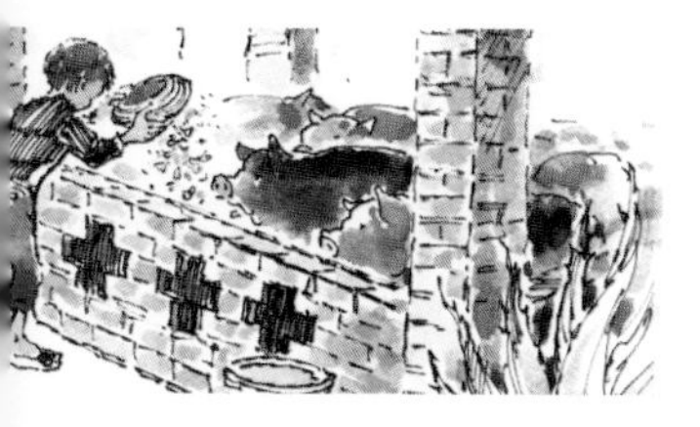

In **Chapter Five** our love of meat has forced science and technology to create extensive applications for animal farming in order to meet our insatiable, meat-centered diet. We will compare these high-protein feeds and commercial, chemically-accelerated grown meats to natural free-range grown meat. At the same time, the question is raised: "Are we animal farming our next generations?"

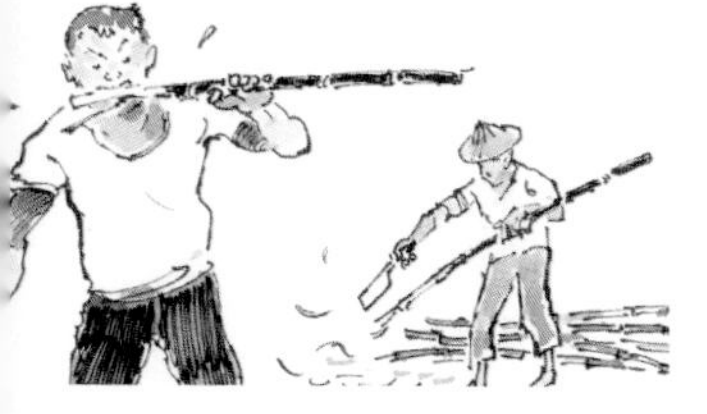

In **Chapter Six** we examine our fondness for sweets. We abuse this pleasure of life, but what can we do about it? Comparing what I have observed today to my childhood's simpler lifestyle in Taiwan, I offer a possible solution.

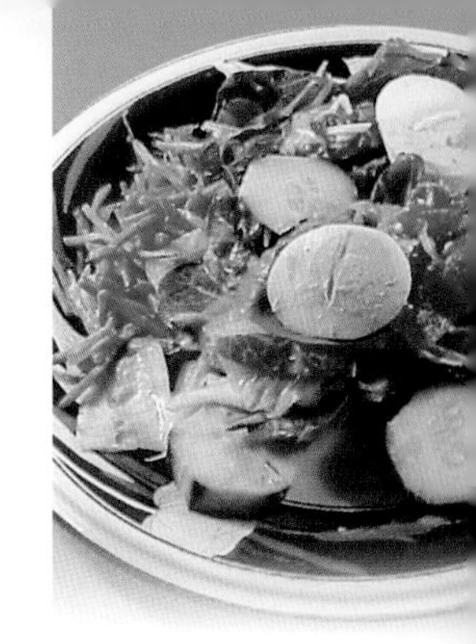

Chapter 4

Salad

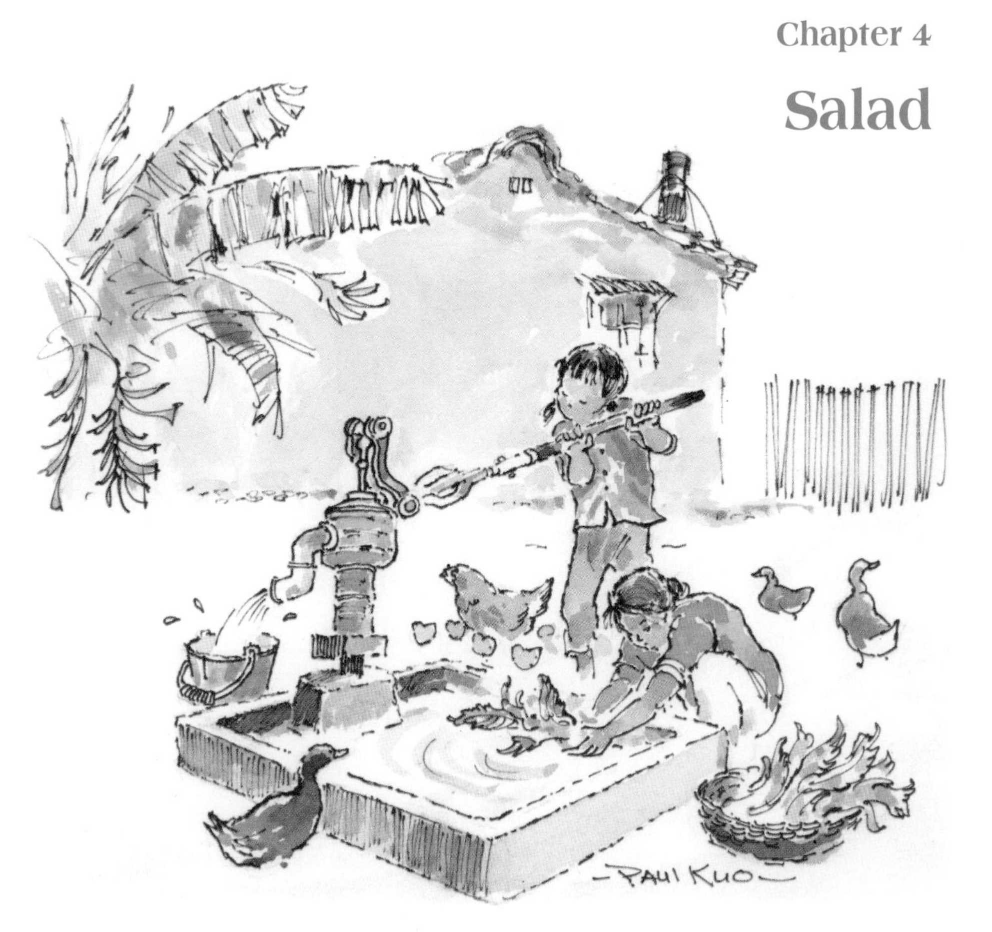

In this section, we discuss the major dietary changes of recent years, changes that may have contributed to some of the problems we face today. It is not my intention for these discussions to be viewed as scare tactics, but only to help readers make informed decisions about their food choices and question presumptions about 'healthy' diets.

Is It Good to Eat Like a Rabbit?

A drastic change in the American diet over the last fifty years has been the growing popularity of raw vegetable salads. Today, when we want to lose weight or improve our health, we immediately think of one food: salad. Salads are an institution as American as apple pie used to be. Salad, usually made of iceberg lettuce, which is high in water-content but low in nutrients, became an integral part of the standard American diet only after chemical fertilizers and insecticides made it possible to grow picture-perfect lettuce consistently. Most restaurant meals include salad as part of the meal and often as the whole meal by itself. And as you know, you can find all-you-can-eat salad bars in restaurants everywhere, even fast-food restaurants.

Popular wisdom tells us that a nice green vegetable salad can provide fiber, vitamins, and the nutrients we need in order to stay healthy, particularly enzymes—the complex group of proteins that catalyze biochemical reactions essential to good health. Dieters especially fall prey to the apparent wisdom of ingesting large portions of salad. Maybe we should examine the merits of salad and its effect on our health from a more critical perspective. Are salads actually as healthy as we have been led to believe?

Raw Versus Cooked Foods

Let's take a close look at the differences between eating raw vegetable salads, including those ever-popular raw veggie-platters that are served with dip and the alternative: cooked vegetables. Along with enzymes, raw vegetables offer an important health benefit—roughage—necessary to eliminate body wastes and toxins. We might also logically assume that eating vegetables raw is the best way to retain the maximum, unspoiled vitamins and nutritional value. However, let's stop and think how our ancestors ate. Archaeological digs have shown, indisputably, that ancient people cooked food, presumably because foods smelled and tasted better when cooked. In fact, researchers believe that early man simply liked the aroma that emanated from cooking.

In the case of vegetables, cooking breaks down the cellulose where nutrients are stored, making cooked foods easier for the body to digest. For example, it is a scientific fact that to get the most beta-carotene (pro-vitamin A) from a carrot, we need to break down its cellular structure. Simply eating the raw, whole carrot provides relatively little quantities of the nutrient to the human body. We can juice or finely grate the carrot, but throughout the ages, most cultures have chosen cooking instead.

Interestingly, various animals eating vegetation as their diet, such as cows and sheep, have four separate stomach chambers for complete digestion. The vegetable foods, usually grass and hay, are

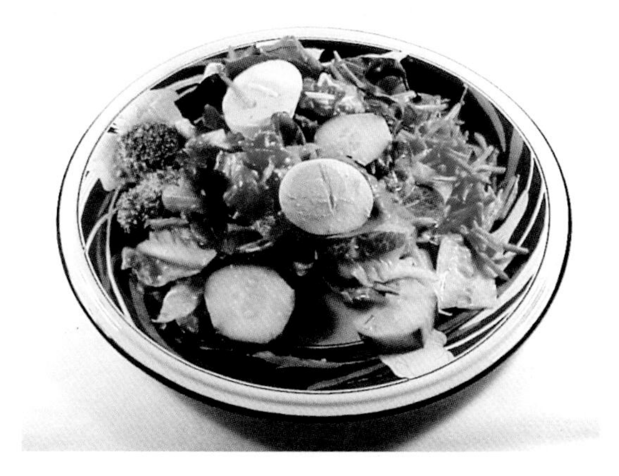

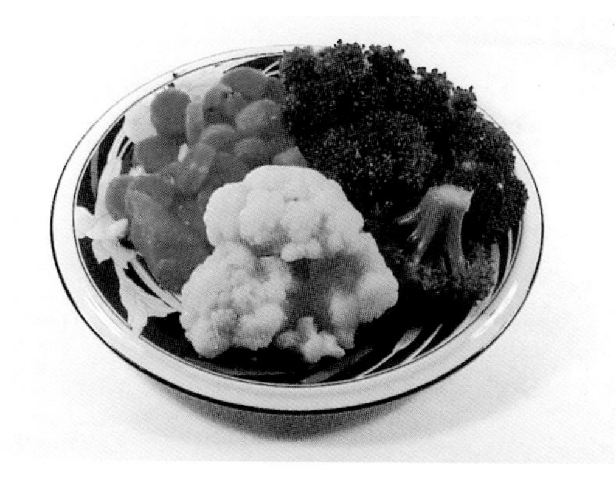

repeatedly regurgitated in one stomach to break them down, and then the naturally processed food mass is transported to a separate stomach for fermentation so the cellulose can be broken down for digestion, a process similar to the effects of cooking. Cooking expedites this process of digestion for humans, whom nature gave only one stomach, fortunately.

As mentioned, we humans are omnivorous, which means we eat all kinds of food, both animal and vegetable. Archaeological evidence shows that throughout the history of the world, most of this food was eaten cooked, not raw, including vegetables.

In many cultures throughout history and, indeed, in most areas of the world today where chemical fertilizers are not available, raw vegetables are considered unsafe because the only fertilizer available is human or animal waste and, to a lesser extent, compost from decayed plant materials. These materials can carry disease from direct contact and ingestion. As a result, cooking food is as necessary to prevent disease as it is to promote good digestion. Let's look even more closely at the advantages of cooking.

Three Reasons Why Foods Need to be Cooked

Parasites and Bacteria

Growing up in Taiwan in the 1950s and 1960s, none of us would even consider eating raw vegetables. The risk of getting sick or infected by parasites was too high. As a matter of fact, in earlier times before the use of chemicals, the British considered fresh vegetables and fruits to be unhealthy because they caused upset stomach and diarrhea. Looking at the past shows us, perhaps surprisingly, that humans have evolved to eat cooked foods and have developed a genetic structure best suited to a mostly-cooked diet.

Even water from the well, which they used to wash the vegetables and to drink, had to be boiled because domesticated animals such as ducks, chickens, and pigs

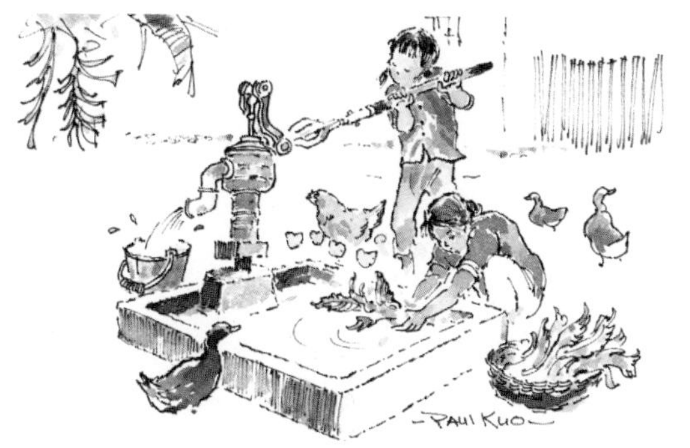

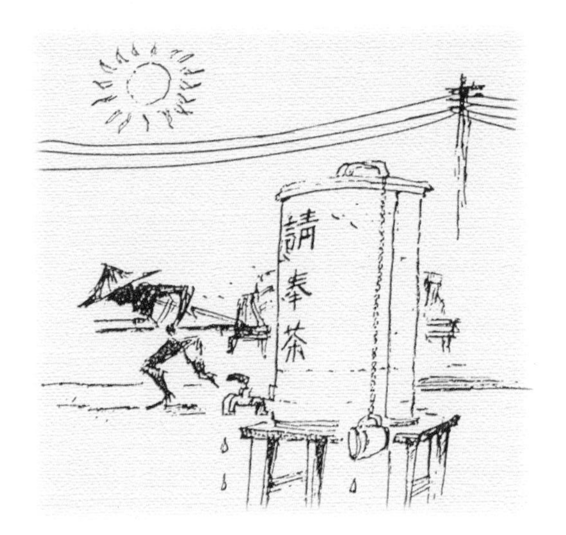

Free tea. The overheated 'pedicab' driver and the sweating pedestrian stop by the roadside for a free drink of tea. No special organization offers this service; it was offered by independent families. In accordance with Buddhist teaching, it is believed that any good deed accrues to the benefit of the benefactor.

roamed the yard, and their waste could easily contaminate the well water. In every household, the first thing mothers did in the morning was to boil drinking water. It was common for a stranger to drop in and ask for a drink of boiled water. Even today, America is one of very few places where people can drink tap water. Drinking boiled water or bottled water is more common throughout most of the rest of the world. If they could afford it, early Britons drank ale instead of water to quench their thirst, and the French drank wine.

Natural Toxins

From another perspective, most living organisms—including plants used for food—have complex defense mechanisms for survival. Built into the chemical structure of plants are certain natural 'pesticides' to help fend off biological enemies, which would include people and the animals that want to eat them, as well as diseases and other predators such as insects, birds, and reptiles. Like all living things, plants produce chemicals so complex that scientists, so far, have been unable to analyze them all. Even though we have advanced technologically in so many ways, we are still incapable of analyzing and understanding the thousands of minute trace chemicals in plants.

For example, some common foods recently tested have been shown to be carcinogenic in trials with lab animals. Recent studies also indicate that the popular alfalfa sprouts may contain canavanine, which can be toxic to humans. Unfortunately, this was only discovered a short time ago, but for a

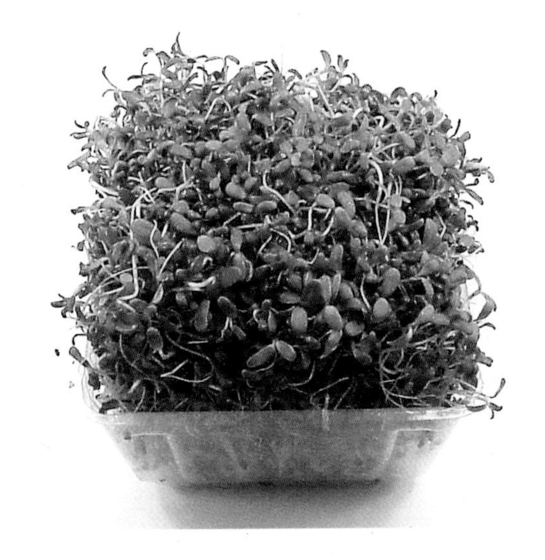

long time, alfalfa sprouts were considered an ideal health food.

So when we eat raw vegetables, including some roots, we are ingesting naturally-occurring chemicals that are part of the plants' protective mechanisms. These chemicals might be harmful to our health, as with alfalfa sprouts. These toxins especially occur in the reproductive parts of the plant to help the species survive.

When we are not eating properly, our bodies can be compromised and our immune systems may be weakened. However, symptoms from these toxins might not be manifested as serious problems for some time. This may be one of the reasons that people have chronic, long-term health problems that our medical professionals can't seem to solve. Our eliminatory organs—the liver, kidneys and so on—must work harder to deal with such food toxins. On the other hand, cooked toxins break down into simpler compounds, which we are genetically adapted to, so we can digest them without harmful effects.

Fruits are a different matter from vegetables. They taste sweet, so humans (and animals) readily eat them and thus spread their seeds through waste elimination, which serves their reproductive purposes. However, the seeds and nuts from fruits, as with vegetables, also contain toxins, usually in the form of digestive inhibitors; that is, they are not broken down in the body but remain whole. So it appears that nature intends for fruit to be eaten as one method of spreading the fruit's seeds. For ideal health, some cooks suggest that you soak nuts and seeds in lightly salted water overnight, and then dry them slowly in a low heated oven. This process enhances the taste while retaining enzyme activity, yet inactivating the inhibitors so that the body can digest them safely.

Plant-eating animals that must rely on raw plant food as their main diet have adapted their digestive systems to neutralize the toxins naturally present. For example, pandas have eaten bamboo leaves and koala bears have eaten eucalyptus leaves as their exclusive diet for ages. Their bodies, through thousands of years of evolution, have developed digestive enzymes to counteract the toxins.

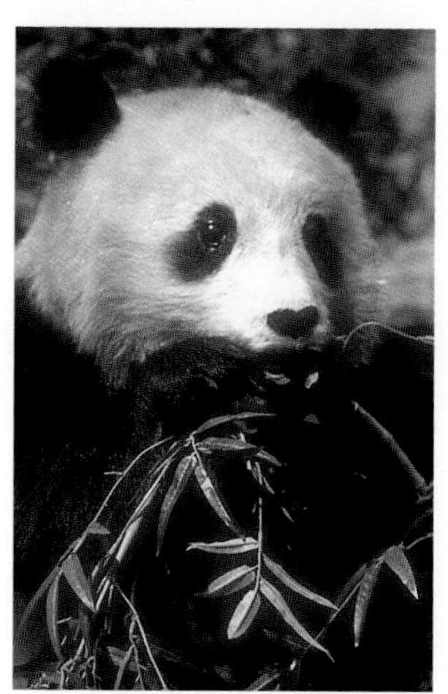

In contrast, we humans don't have this ability to neutralize raw food toxins. When people begin a raw foods diet, they may feel good at first because of the infusion of enzymes and the lightness of the food. After a time, however, their bodies can't handle the cumulative effect, their body's ability to fend off the toxins may be diminished, and their health deteriorates. Children in families enforcing a raw-foods regimen may fail to develop robustly, and these children often suffer tooth decay and poor bone formation. Generally, over the long term, people on raw foods diets suffer from stunted growth or disproportionate body shape, crooked teeth, bowed legs, dull hair, cracked nails, and more.

Pesticides and Chemicals

The mainstay of salad is tender, green leaves, mostly lettuce, whether iceberg or other varieties. To grow these commercially, farmers have to use pesticides to keep the greens safe from insect damage. Since these tender leaves have such high water content, they are especially attractive to insects; therefore, growers must apply chemicals. Spinach or romaine lettuce with noticeable insect holes will not sell in the grocery stores or be accepted in any restaurant. Requiring a perfect cosmetic appearance of produce has led to an overuse of pesticides.

This is yet another reason why cooking is so fundamental: when we cook vegetables, the heat vaporizes the chemicals and reduces their concentration drastically. When heated, the chemicals generally break down to be less complex, which results in less toxic compounds, or else they simply evaporate. And of course, after cooking vegetables, we don't have to worry about infectious diseases from human handling being transmitted on the leaves.

Recent reports indicate that, contrary to popular belief, American produce contains more excessive pesticides and chemicals than the produce imported from South America. Carefully washing and cooking the vegetables to minimize chemical intake is about all we can do unless we want to pay the higher prices for organically-grown vegetables.

Playing the Hand that Nature Dealt Us

It is clear that our ancestors did not eat uncooked vegetables and, therefore, it is logical to assume that our genetic structure does not provide the ability to easily digest raw foods and optimally absorb their nutrients. Our bodies simply lack the ability to neutralize the undesirable, natural toxic compounds in raw vegetables.

There is ample evidence that our bodies function best if we eat foods similar to what our ancestors ate. In other words, we need to play the hand that nature dealt us. For instance, most Asians cannot tolerate dairy products. Many African Americans and American Indians have the same problem. They lack the lactase enzyme required to digest milk products properly. Obviously, such people should just forego or minimize dairy products. So far, no one has scientifically proven the idea that our genetic inheritance directly affects our digestion, and it is impossible to conduct clinical trials on such things.

Salad consumption is relatively new; it became an important part of our diet only after the use of agricultural chemicals became widespread. Many of our unexplained medical problems began about the same time, and I do not think this is mere coincidence.

For some of us, totally giving up raw vegetable salads may be too hard. We should at least consider washing our raw vegetables in a water solution of salt and vinegar; that is, one or more teaspoons of salt and the same amount of vinegar in a quart of water. This adds a little salty flavor to the vegetables and may reduce the bacterial count and, at the same time, it may help neutralize some of the toxic chemicals present on the vegetables.

Recently published research indicates that our bodies digest and absorb cooked vegetables much better than uncooked vegetables. Lightly cooking vegetables retains most of the benefits of raw vegetable salads (such as fiber and vitamins) and minimizes, or eliminates, most of the negative effects.

Many vegetables cannot be eaten raw; they can be outright poisonous if not cooked or, at the very least, have a disagreeable taste, but they can become a healthy delicious dish after cooking. A good example of this is artichokes. It is also easy to season vegetables and enhance their flavor when cooking them. What we need to know is how to cook vegetables properly and eat them in a way that maximizes their benefit while retaining a pleasurable taste.

Remember Fermented Foods

To get the benefit of eating raw vegetables, traditional cultures around the world have come up with a very effective technique: fermentation. Pickling vegetables uses fermentation, which preserves the vegetables by taking advantage of the beneficial effects of lactobacillus bacteria. Just about every culture has some form of 'pickles.' These are very different from the

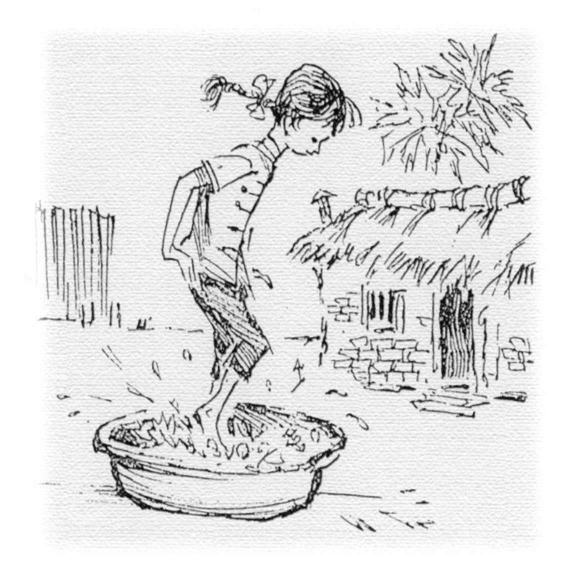

Homely custom. Shredded radish is put into a tub to be trampled with salt. The mixture is then dried in the sun to make a condiment noted for its ability to whet the appetite. Quite a feat.

vinegar pickles that we can buy in supermarkets today. Instead, vegetables are preserved by lacto-fermentation, which is a natural way of preserving foods. I say that it's natural because the lactobacillus bacteria, which occur everywhere in nature, are responsible for this type of fermentation. Starches and sugars in vegetables and fruits are converted into lactic acid by these bacteria that are present on the surface of all living things, especially on the leaves and roots of plants growing in or near the ground. Most cultures the world over have their variations on this theme: sauerkraut, as well as pickled cucumbers, beets and turnips in Europe; pickled green tomatoes, peppers, and lettuce in Russia and Poland; and the wide variety of pickled vegetables eaten in the Orient including Japan, China, and Korea.

If you dine in a Korean restaurant, you will be served a side dish of *kim chi*, a hot and spicy fermented cabbage dish. Typically, these fermented foods are served as small side dishes consumed to help enhance digestion, which includes supplying enzymes for digestion and overall good health. Similarly, in Taiwan, preserved raw foods are usually eaten with every meal. These may include pickled cabbage, cucumbers, leafy greens, daikon radishes, and bean curd (tofu).

A traditional Taiwanese breakfast, usually a light meal, consists of soupy rice with preserved veggies. As in cultures around the world, these Taiwanese pickles are salty and tasty—and fermented. The vegetables used for this process are commonly presented as a free side dish together with hot tea in most respectable Chinese restaurants as well. It is very easy to pickle heavy, rich leaves and roots, as opposed to the light and tender leaves you might commonly see in salads. I describe in detail how to make these dishes in Chapter Twelve, and I invite you to try them.

During a recent trip to Europe, I noticed that most small village restaurants serve, as appetizers, a plate of pickled foods to whet the appetite. We were almost always served such a plate in Italy.

The fermentation, as well as the sour and salty taste of the pickled vegetables, stimulates the secretion of saliva to aid digestion and nutrient absorption. At the end of the meal, we were often served a small piece of fruit such as an orange or a piece of watermelon. This fruit adds more enzymes, which again act as a catalyst to help the body digest the food. Similarly, in many cultures, people enjoyed an after-dinner drink and a piece of cheese. Traditional people—our ancestors—did not know about enzymes but, over time, they concluded that certain foods eaten at mealtime could help digestion and overall health.

Eat Veggies for Your Health

We all agree that eating our veggies is absolutely vital to good health, but the question here is *how* we eat vegetables. There are so many different varieties of veggies available, with very few of them included in our raw veggie salads. The popularity of eating raw salads over the last few decades has almost made us forget how to cook our veggies. We can just pop a veggie bag into the microwave now without a second thought. Today, the popular methods of cooking vegetables, such as boiling and microwaving, result in vegetable dishes that are bland and predictable, not particularly delicious, as well as quite restrictive in variety. Your kids, no doubt, let you know how unsatisfying this is! To improve the flavor, we add butter or mayonnaise. But the end result is that cooked veggies have become less and less important in our daily fare. To improve our diet, the first priority is to learn how to cook vegetables.

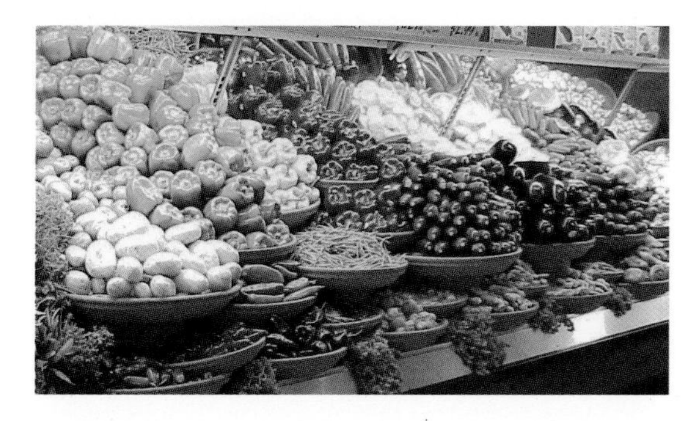

The Chinese method of stir-fry may be an effective way of reintroducing vegetables into our diet. Simple and practical, stir-frying has served the Chinese well for generations. Chinese cooking has developed and evolved for over five thousand years of long and continuous civilization. People often mistakenly think it is a complex, sophisticated, and difficult way to prepare food. Overall, judging from the popularity of Chinese restaurants all over America, Chinese cooking is well accepted by the American population. In recent years, Chinese buffets have been springing up all over the country. Americans are learning that Chinese stir-fry is actually great for everyday eating, but how to stir-fry remains a daunting task for many of us.

In this book, I propose a modified way of preparing stir-fry—as well as other dishes—that is simple and easy to adapt into our modern kitchens and lifestyles; yet it is flexible enough to allow us to eat all kinds of veggies, properly prepared and delicious, so our bodies can digest and absorb their nutrients. Using these techniques, anybody can prepare a wholesome, healthy meal in as little time as it might take to go out for fast-food. With a little preparation and some experimenting, I think you will be pleasantly surprised at how easy it is to cook this way and expand on the variety of veggies you consume.

As we make changes to fit our modern life, we have abandoned very important aspects of our traditions to the detriment of our health. These changes have happened almost without our knowing it. One generation gives up traditional foods for more popular fare, and their children never learn to eat the way their ancestors did for generations to come. In Part Four, I offer simple techniques for preparing and cooking foods to help you and your family rediscover the traditional roots of your ancestors.

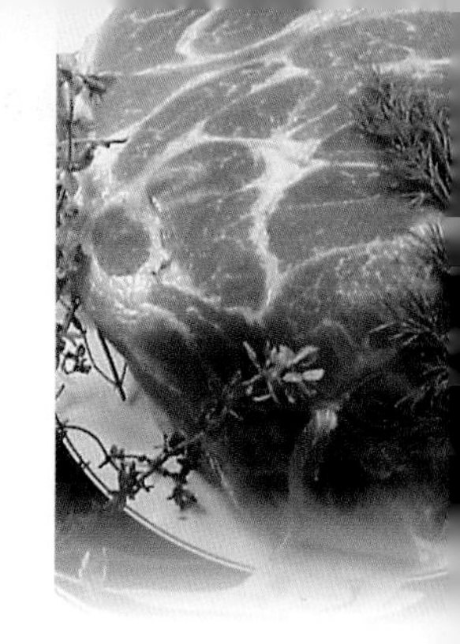

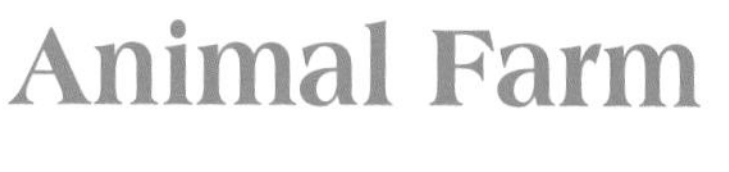

Chapter 5
Animal Farm

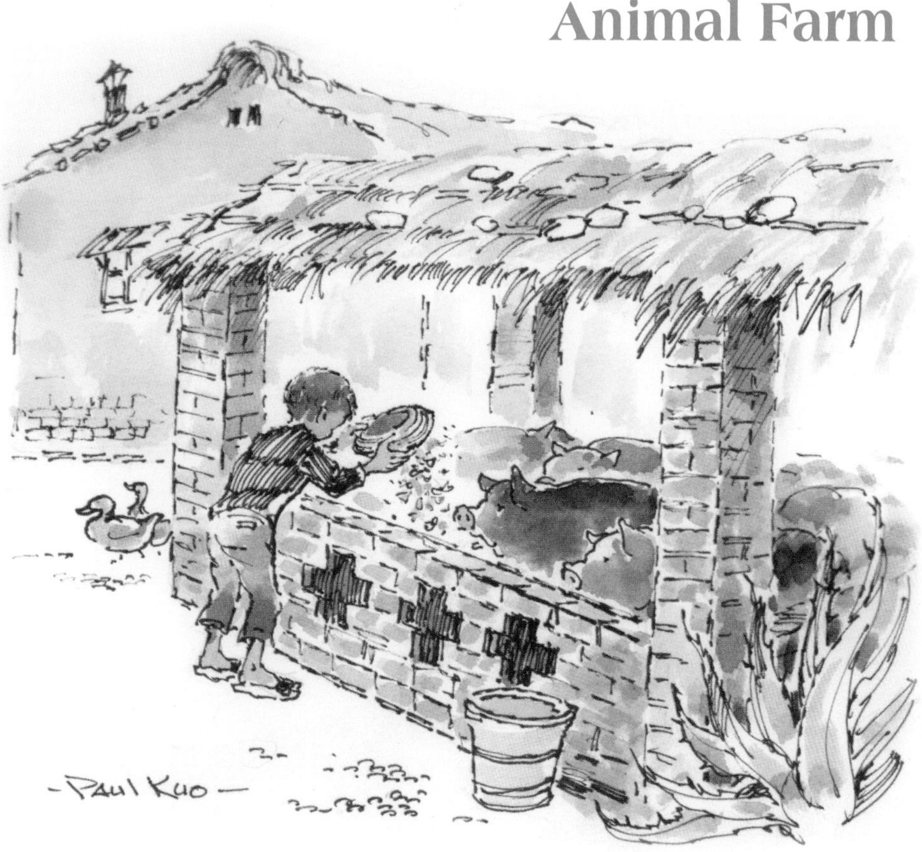

In addition to raw vegetable salads, one other significant change in the American diet since the turn of the twentieth century is how much meat we eat. While most traditional cultures build their diets around grains and vegetables, we Americans usually base our meals on meat with other foods added for variety.

As Americans, we inherited, through the English culture, a love of meat. Also, the prosperity of post-war years, including high-tech animal farming, has made it easy to indulge in excessive amounts of meat in our diets, which may be adversely affecting our health.

Grains Are for People

I grew up in a small village in Taiwan, an island with many mountains and limited land for agriculture. We were lucky to be in the tropical zone (the Tropic of Cancer actually passes through the middle of Taiwan), so the weather is good for growing food.

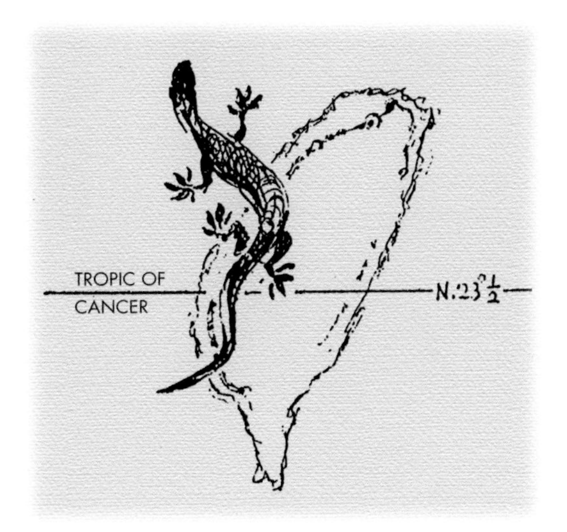

Wall lizard. No home should be without a few of these friendly fellows. The Taipei variety is positively silent. The Taichung type emits an occasional disapproving "Tsk, tsk!" But South of Chiayi and, the Tropic of Cancer, they become really vocal, "Geck, geck, gecko." Why? No one knows.

Most of us were far from wealthy, so our diet was simple, typical of most traditional cultures. Our staple foods were rice, sweet potatoes, and vegetables, but not a great deal of meat. Each farmer had a working water buffalo (or two) to help with the farming, and much of the meat we had—pigs, chickens, ducks—we raised ourselves in our yards. You could see them just about everywhere; in fact, they looked like pets instead of farm animals.

Most people raised pigs because a pig will eat just about anything. They can convert most leftovers and waste from food preparation, such as the trimmings and peelings from vegetables, into meat. Grains were an important staple food for people and considered too expensive to feed animals. Until you've raised pigs, you don't really know the meaning of the expression, "Eats like a pig."

Early before sunrise every day, we could hear a pig squealing on the way to the slaughterhouse, its feet bound together, hanging on a bamboo pole slung between two men. Walking to school in the morning, we could see the pieces of the slaughtered pig hanging by the feet at the butcher's stand. Every part of the animal was prepared for use, including the internal organs and blood. By early afternoon, the whole animal was sold. We were a village of several hundred people, but one pig slaughtered per day supplied an adequate amount of meat to the entire

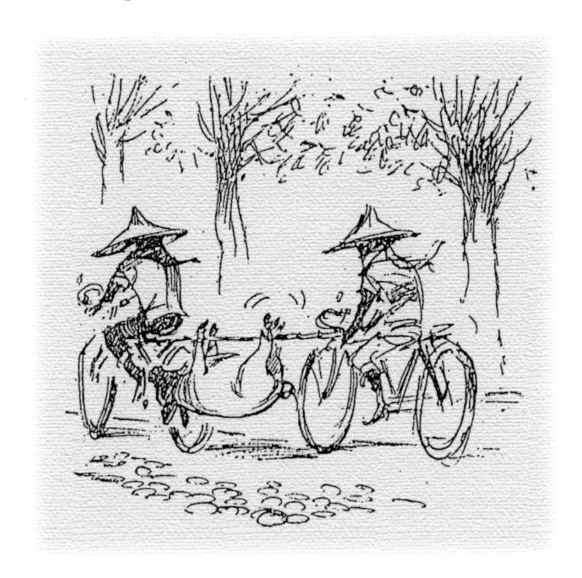

To market, to market. Oink, oink! This porker got a little too hefty, so it took two farmer acrobats to cart him off to slaughter. But he had his hour of glory as a prime porker.

village, except for special holidays when more than one pig was killed. Special occasions, such as a visit from an important visitor or a holiday, might also call for the slaughter of a chicken or duck from one of the family's flock.

We considered meat to be somewhat of a luxury. We often ate meat with our meals, but only in small amounts. We cut it into small pieces and cooked it with vegetables so everybody got some and felt satisfied with the meal. Using meat this way—almost like a garnish, not the main event—is typical in most traditional cultures.

Our Abundant Meat Supply

In 1962, when I arrived in California as a student, I roomed with five other students in a house. Each roommate cooked his own meals. I was shocked at the amount of meat and milk products my American roommates ate every day. I had never had a pork chop or steak back home; in fact, I had never even seen one before, since in our cooking, we didn't use meat so generously! I could not believe that anyone would eat such a big piece of meat at one meal. When I went to the supermarket, I was impressed with how much meat was there for sale. The meat was carefully prepared and packaged so it didn't even look like it came from an animal. It also tasted slightly different from what we had back home. That's when I became curious about how meats were produced in the United States.

Animals As Machines that Convert Grain to Meat

In 1995, at a tennis event in Maui, I met John, the owner of a poultry company near Jackson, Mississippi. John told me that in his poultry plant, they processed 20,000 chickens per *hour*, and the production line was open for sixteen hours a day with the remaining eight hours used to sanitize the facility. So in reality, the plant was open twenty-four hours a day all year round. Do a simple calculation: this single plant processes 320,000 chickens a day.

On the average, each chicken weighs five to six pounds; two pounds of feed are needed to produce one pound of chicken. Thus, the plant slaughtered approximately 1.5 million pounds of chicken produced from 3 million pounds of chicken feed per day. These numbers may seem astronomical, and we might think that this was an enormous poultry plant; yet according to John, his plant was a small operation; most others in the area were larger.

On an impulse, I asked John if I could come and visit his poultry plant, and he graciously agreed. One nice, warm, spring day the following year, we visited John's poultry plant in Mississippi. Our guide during the visit was Dr. Wang, a Ph.D. from Texas A&M, and an expert in nutrition.

We started the tour at the egg hatchery. Every egg hatched out in twenty-one days. A conveyer belt moved the newly hatched chicks constantly into a room where workers stood on both sides of the line and gave each chick a shot of vaccine.

Next, the belt moved the chicks across a counter and pushed them into a basket, 200 chicks to the basket. Then 20,000 chicks were transported in one truck to a chicken growing facility where all the feed and water were automatically supplied. The chicks lived in the minimum space to keep them alive without much room to move around. The air was constantly circulated, but the nasty smell of decaying chicken droppings permeated the air in and around the entire facility.

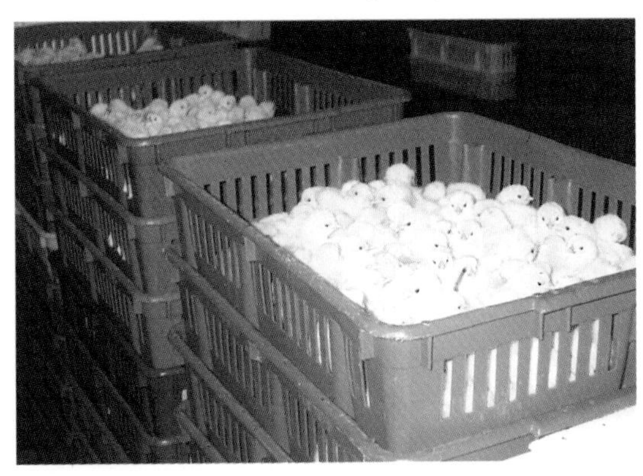

Hundreds of chicks per basket on a production line.

The feed was constantly monitored for optimal growth at each stage of the chicken's life. As you would expect, most of the feed was a combination of grains, but new technology added a protein component. Since certain parts of the chicken are not marketable, such as blood, feet, heads, and feathers, these high-protein chicken parts were processed and reused as part of the feed. In addition, chemicals were added to accelerate growth or prevent disease.

Of course, a certain percentage of the chicks die, especially in hot summer weather. Nevertheless, in only forty-two to fifty days, a tiny chick became a six-pound chicken. Since these chicks were only forty-two days old when slaughtered, by any standards, they were still baby chicks that weighed six pounds. In human terms, these chicks would be considered clinically obese youngsters!

Spurred on by my curiosity about meat production, on other occasions, I visited a deer farm in New Zealand and a shrimp and eel farm in Taiwan.

They all shared one overriding concern: how much feed does it take to grow a pound of meat, and how fast can you do it? In fish farming, I was told that one pound of feed would grow one pound of fish, which results in the most efficient conversion of feed to meat. It takes

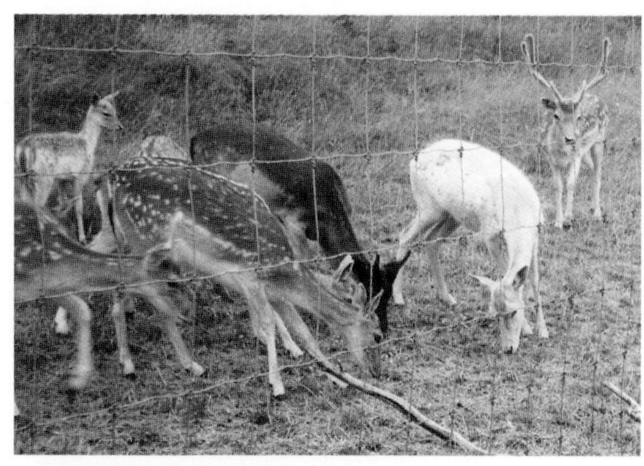
A deer farm I visited in New Zealand.

high protein feed made from grains and other ingredients to accomplish this. Of course, chemicals are added to the feed for disease control and accelerated growth. These meat growers have it down to a precise science.

Because we have plenty of grain in America, coupled with a highly developed technology, we have plenty to feed to our animals so there's an abundance of affordable meat to supply our ever-more-affluent population. Today, with our reliance on fast-food restaurants (mostly beef hamburgers and chicken) and our love of meat-dominated dinners, American meat consumption has reached an extremely high level, a certain prescription for health problems.

In mass production animal farming, we treat animals like machines that simply convert grain to meat. The chickens we saw on the farms were like zombies; they showed little or no reaction to any outside stimuli. The workers treated them like a piece of lifeless meat even though they were still alive. The only reason they came into this world was to grow into an obese youngster in the shortest amount of time. Of course, to produce a chicken, you need to have chicks, which come easily from eggs.

On hog farms, to produce a baby piglet is another story. Mother pigs are chemically stimulated to produce piglets in large quantities, and they are fertilized by artificial insemination. The sole purpose of a mother pig's existence is to produce piglets. She is like a piggy-producing machine; so she's big and fat and can barely move. Through chemistry and technology, she produces many more babies than a normal pig could possibly produce, and the piglets she produces are genetically engineered to grow as fast as possible.

Natural Ways to Raise Animals

In contrast, back home in Taiwan, most families kept a few pigs to consume leftovers—sort of like a living garbage disposal—and turn them into meat. They were fed foods that were unacceptable to humans. If they were ever fed grain, it was spoiled, low quality products. They grew lean and at a slower pace.

When a sow was in estrus, she was impregnated by a boar owned by a stud service—

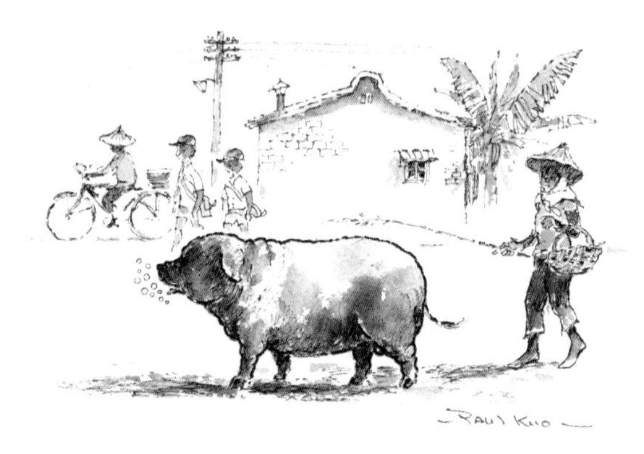

usually a boar owned by an old lady in the neighborhood. This lucky sire followed the lady from village to village every day to visit the eligible sows.

Every once in a while, we could see the old lady and the boar travel together as we walked to school in the morning. Believe me, we could smell them as they got close. As youngsters, we were permitted to watch the whole mating process. Our parents probably thought it was easier for us to watch pigs mate than to teach us the story of the birds and the bees.

This sire performed his job very professionally. In just minutes, he was on his way home. In a few months, about ten piglets were born. The piglets were nursed for the natural amount of time. When they were hungry, all of them came squealing and begging to be fed. The mother pig would lie down, making her special call of "come and get it!" Without a doubt, these pigs behaved like the intelligent, living animals that they are.

Most families on Taiwan also kept chickens and ducks in their yards. Ducks liked to play and feed where it was wet, while chickens ran around the yards surrounding our homes. They were constantly pecking and feeding from the ground. Hens typically lay one egg each day for a couple of weeks and then get ready to hatch the eggs by sitting on the nest. When a hen got broody, or 'clucky,' that is, ready to sit on a clutch of eggs, she'd sit on a nest with or without eggs.

If our mother decided that we didn't need any more baby chicks, we could eat the eggs. As a kid, I loved to eat fresh, raw egg. When a hen laid an egg, she cackled triumphantly and jumped off the nest. We picked up the egg, cracked it, and ate it raw. There were never any reports of people getting sick from eating raw eggs.

A hen might produce between twelve and sixteen eggs, which were allowed to

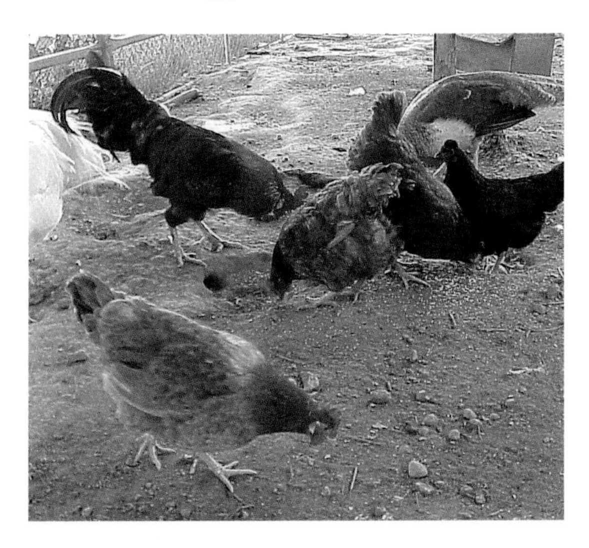

hatch out in about twenty-one days. Mother hens are very good mothers. They take all the chicks and walk them around in the yard. If they find food, they call the chicks with a special cluck to come and get it. If we threw a handful of grain on the ground, the mother hen guarded it until the chicks were fed. If she saw an eagle or hawk, she clucked wildly to warn the chicks so they could come and hide under her wing.

Ducks and geese are also very protective; they will even attack people to protect their young if they feel threatened. Any dog that hurt or ate a chicken or duck was not allowed to live in the village. The poultry were fed once a day, mostly with rice hulls or other grain-based foods that the family would not eat. Sometimes, we children were sent into the fields to pick some weeds for the ducks and geese. Their favorite food was earthworms; they dug around the yard and fields to find them. Every evening before sunset, they all gathered cooperatively in a spot for us to place them in a protective cage.

Chickens are harder to raise than ducks or geese because they catch diseases so easily. On the other hand, like pigs, ducks or geese will eat just about anything, and they are easier to maintain.

Recently, I bought four duck eggs to hatch so my grandchildren could see what an egg is actually for. They watched the baby ducklings peck their way out of the eggshell, and then a few hours after they were born, the baby ducks started to eat. By the third day, they ate whatever we gave them—table scraps, restaurant leftovers, and kitchen scraps, including vegetable and fruit peels. These ducks grew very fast; at first, they almost doubled their size every two days. It's a wonderful way for nature to turn our food scraps into a meal.

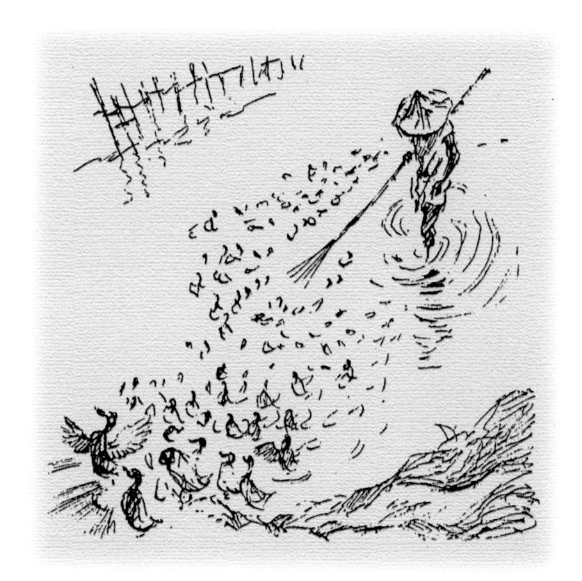

Duck herder. It takes a patient man to ride herd on this bunch of quacks all day long. Shallow rivers and fallow paddies are favorite spots for keeping ducks. Sooner or later they wind up on the table.

Chickens can be quite intuitive and sensitive. When the time came for them to become a dish on the table, they could sense it and often got very nervous, alert, and sometimes went into hiding. Mother killed them in private, out of view of the youngsters. Following Buddhist teachings, she would say a prayer, "We have to kill you to sustain our life. I will pray for you so in your next life you will be born as a human and will not be killed and eaten." Unlike the chicken farm, where chickens are slaughtered at maximum economic value of about six to seven weeks old, in Taiwan we killed the chickens when they reached sexual maturity at about three or four months old. Traditional Chinese medicine taught that matured meat has more 'chi' and so is better for our body.

Did You Ever Try Beijing Duck?

Most Americans aren't familiar with duck meat, which has a stronger taste than other poultry. You need to know how to cook duck to make it taste good. The most famous way to prepare duck is Beijing duck, which Americans came to know through Henry Kissinger during his initial Open Door visit to China in the late 1970s. Roasted ducks, which hang on the window of barbeque deli stores in Chinatown, taste almost the same as Beijing duck, if not better. The barbecued ducks are very inexpensive, something worth trying if you ever get to Chinatown. As a matter of fact, in America, we have high quality ducks that are superior to those you will find in Beijing.

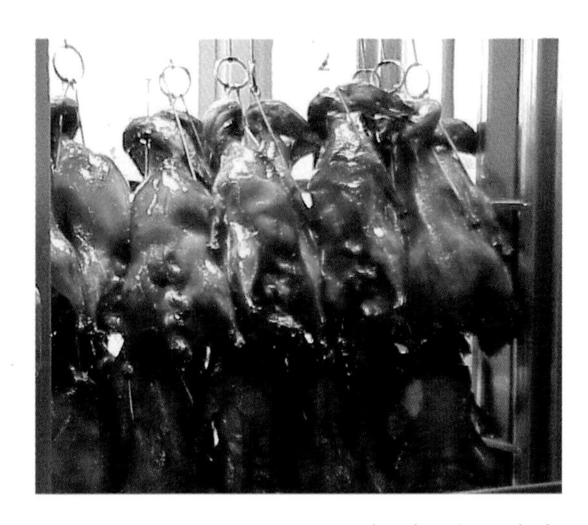

In serving Beijing Duck, the first dish is skin only. The skin of the duck has a nice crispy texture and flavor, and makes a tasty sandwich with tortilla-like steamed bread, served with plum sauce and green onions. The meat and bones are then served as another dish or made into a delicious soup.

Naturally Grown Meat Versus High-Tech Meat

As you can see, the natural way of producing meat is very different from meat produced through high-tech farming. Naturally grown meat is firmer and tastier, and takes longer to cook. The high-tech farm meat tastes mushy and less flavorful. It is not difficult to find out why. High-tech farming mixes special feed with chemicals to stimulate growth rate, control diseases, and produce high-weight animals. A chicken grown naturally and fed on low protein feed, grows at a much slower rate, and the meat is leaner and more mature. Newcomers to this country can tell the difference right away.

Today, in many cities where there is a Chinatown, poultry stores sell live, farm-raised chickens and ducks. Customers choose which chicken or duck they want, and the storekeeper cleans it and sells it, head and feet included. We pay a price for freshness and for the natural meat, but I think it does taste considerably better. Few modern Americans have experienced the taste of fresh, farm-raised chicken, but with experience, you can certainly tell the difference.

Unfortunately, it is almost impossible for us to have meat harvested from lean, free-range poultry, free of chemical hormones and antibiotics—the kinds of meat our bodies are genetically programmed to digest. Instead, most of us grow up eating factory-farmed meat from genetically altered animals whose sole purpose is to grow fat and fast to satisfy our meat-craving appetite. That's the price we pay for more affordable meat. However, if you ever get the chance to eat meat grown naturally from a small farm, don't pass it up!

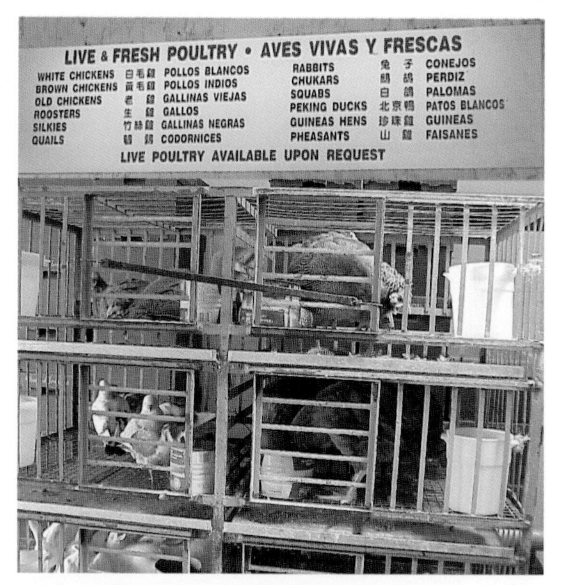

Fresh poultry store in Chinatown. The list is in English, Chinese, and Spanish. Newcomers from South America are important customers.

Meat As Part of a Balanced Meal

Having this inexpensive meat available has made the fast-food and processed food industries grow enormously as well. What can we do about it? To begin with, high-tech meat may not be as wholesome, but it tastes good, and it has the nutrients of naturally grown meat. It is affordable and we should enjoy it, but we should not abuse it by over-consuming.

This is the main point of my stories and observations: cheap meat is no more beneficial to us than cheap wine if consumed in excess and out of balance with other nutritious foods. It just takes becoming aware of the problem and knowing how to manage it. We should simply reduce our meat consumption by modifying our dietary habits. Instead of a meat-centered dinner (like chicken or roast beef) that overloads our body with meat products, we can change the way we prepare our foods and offer meat as a garnish in vegetable dishes. We need a certain amount of protein, of course, but certainly not as much as we Americans typically eat.

How can we reduce the amount of meat we eat? First of all, it takes a different approach to meat preparation. It's not hard to learn the basic skills for preparing a healthy meal, and these skills will last for a lifetime. In the latter part of this book, I present a simple and easy technique to prepare delicious meals combining meat and vegetables. Reducing the amount of meat intake and complementing meat with other balanced nutrients is the best we can do under present circumstances.

Are We Animal Farming Our Babies?

The realities of American animal farming really come home when we think about feeding babies and children. I wonder how much difference there really is between human and animal nutritional science. After all, most of the studies conducted for *human* nutritional science are based on animal research. The biology and nutritional science for animals and humans are similar. If we are not careful, without realizing it, we may be raising our babies in a way that is similar to methods used on modern animal farms. Let me give you just one prime example.

Nature provides mothers with breast milk for babies. For thousands of years, mother's milk was the natural and normal way to take care of infants; it never occurred to people that breast-feeding could be obscene or unnatural. In modern times, many municipalities actually passed ordinances prohibiting breast-feeding in public since women's breasts had taken on a predominantly sexual connotation. But women have breast-fed their babies from the beginning of time!

After some months, when an infant starts to get bigger and his first baby teeth appear, mothers begin to wean their babies and gradually introduce them to solid food.

Over the last fifty years, however, food companies have worked hard to convince

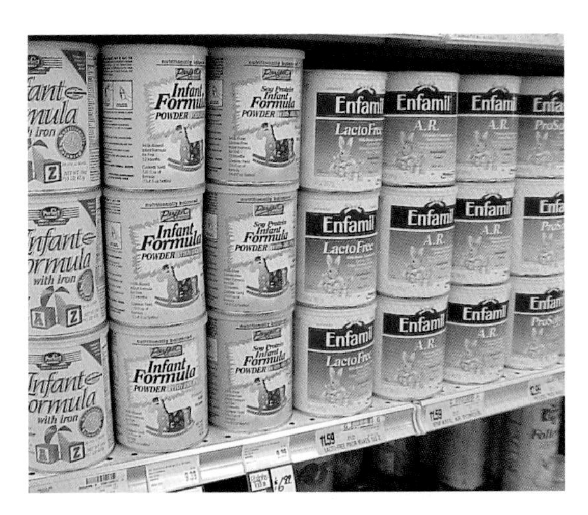

us that this traditional way of feeding babies could be improved. Baby formula was invented to replace natural milk. Today, we are often told that what our mothers or grandmothers did was backward and unscientific, and that it interferes with our modern lifestyle. To grow healthy babies, the formula companies imply that we should feed them scientifically.

What Is Baby Formula?

How are baby formulas created? The answer may surprise you. They are based on the same nutritional science we use to produce animal feed. Dr. Wang—the Ph.D. from Texas A&M who accompanied our tour through the poultry plant—could work for a baby formula company and perform the same kind of work he does with the poultry industry. Look at the label of a can of baby formula. The long, complex list of ingredients is printed there, but unless you have a Ph.D. in nutritional science, there's no way you can figure out what all these ingredients are.

We assume that formulas contain all the nutrients a baby needs. In addition, chemicals are added to make the formula look good, smell good, and mix up easily. But common sense tells us that no formula can ever be the same as natural mother's milk. It does not look or smell like mother's milk: mother's milk looks thin and blue compared to formula. It is naïve to believe our babies get the same or better nutrients from this processed imitation. Mother's milk changes over the months, as the baby's nutritional needs change, and no formula can duplicate this. It also contains enzymes for its digestion and antibodies from the mother's system to help protect the baby from disease. Fortunately, there is a trend back to breast-feeding in this country.

So from birth, many American babies begin their lives by consuming food that is 'engineered' and processed. By the time these babies can talk, television bombards them with relentless propaganda to program them to eat commercially processed foods. One step at a time, this brainwashing process continues for the rest of the child's impressionable years. Over the last five decades, a minuscule grain of sand in the hourglass of human history, we have changed our diet from eating natural, unrefined foods to eating processed foods, starting from infancy.

In the last fifty years, our whole American lifestyle has changed drastically. We have invented everything from airplanes to penicillin; we have invented the nuclear bomb. We have seen a multitude of medical advances, and great changes in nutritional science, and with all that change, our diet and lifestyle have changed as well. And not for the better.

Chicken Breasts Grown on Chicken Trees

Today, our food arrives so well packaged with plastic that many of us don't even know where it comes from. It is almost as though we are conditioned to think that chicken breasts grow on a chicken tree, and all a chicken farmer has to do is pick one off the tree. Does that sound outrageous?

One year on April Fool's Day, the British Broadcasting Company (BBC) aired a program showing spaghetti farmers harvesting spaghetti from a tree. The tree was hung full of spaghetti. The reporter talked about the favorable weather conditions that year resulting in a good crop of spaghetti. There were surprising numbers of people who believed the story. I would bet that most people you meet have never actually picked an apple from a tree, much less gathered fresh eggs from a hen's nest. I am certain that most people have never seen an animal slaughtered for meat.

Like it or not, today most of us live a fairly artificial lifestyle. We can't easily change the whole thing, but we can be wise in the way we live. When we have babies, for example, we can choose to breast-feed them instead of giving formula, especially during the first few months. We can feed our children home-baked snacks instead of processed, commercial products, and accustom them to eating fruits and other natural foods.

We are fortunate to live in this time and place, which provides us with the good life. On the other hand, we can recognize and be aware of some of the deficiencies that exist and try to improve them. As we do this, we'll make our good lives even better.

❖ ❖ ❖

Chapter 6
Sweets

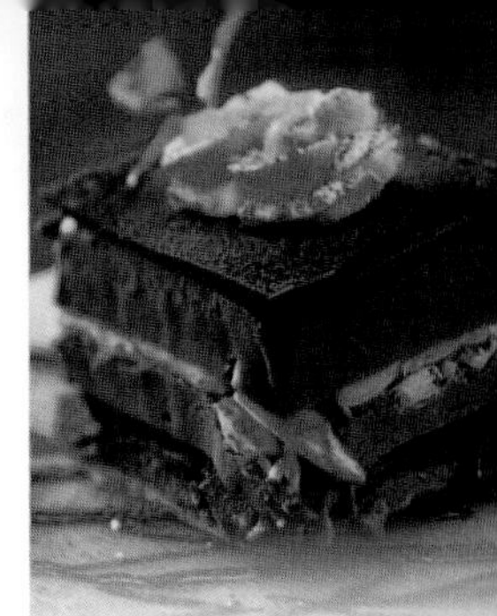

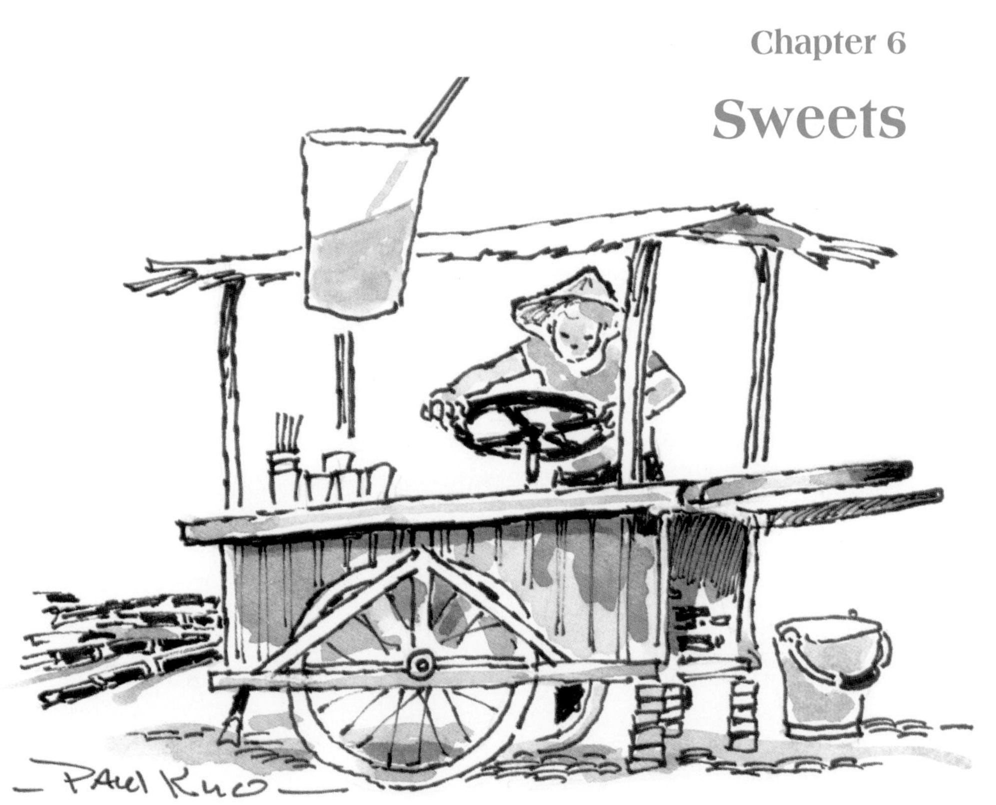

You are familiar with the old expression, "Too much of a good thing." The way we overuse sugar is a great example of this. During most of the history of mankind, we have loved sugar or sweets. In the old days, sugar was too expensive for most people to buy. Introduced from India into Persia around 700 A.D. as a spice, it was the end of the eleventh century before sugar reached the countries of northwestern Europe.

Where Does Sugar Come From?

Although the sugar of early days was very different than the highly-refined sugar we know today, it was still somewhat refined. Pieces of sugarcane were cut into short lengths, crushed, and then pressed to get the juice out. This juice was poured into long, flat pans and gently simmered, the same as evaporating seawater to get sea salt. Once it thickened enough, it was poured into molds to cool and harden. Boiling evaporated the water and separated out the organic matter, which was skimmed off, so the more the sugar was boiled, the more concentrated it became. If people wanted more refined sugar, they boiled it several more times. Each time the sugar was boiled, it became more concentrated, sweeter, and more expensive.

Sugar was mostly used as medicine, thought to be good for colds and for consumption (the old term for tuberculosis). In fact, for the Romans, sugar was *only* used as medicine. The least-refined sugar was sold in large loaves of various sizes. These sugar loaves had much of the original, organic material in them, still somewhat crude, so at the middle of the sugar loaf was a core of dark, impure crystals, brown or almost black. This early sugar had all the natural nutrients and was not nearly as sweet as modern sugar.

Refined sugar is a pure chemical substance of non-nutritive, empty calories that rob the body of vitamins and minerals.

After the English colonized islands in the Caribbean, sugar was both easy to produce and plentiful, so European and British consumers began to demand finer and sweeter grades of it. Consequently, many sugar refineries appeared in London and at major British seaports. The coarse sugar was first boiled with lye made from ashes or lime, which were skimmed off to separate out the impurities. Then the skimmed syrup was clarified with egg whites and further processed to become fine-grade sugar. This was poured into loaves like the less-refined raw sugar, but still did not produce the same crystal white sugar like we have today.

The rich purchased it by the loaf, which weighed perhaps a few pounds, but the poor could buy only a few ounces scraped from the loaf, which was weighed out onto a piece of paper. A pound of sugar was worth a full day's wage for an average craftsman.

During the Elizabethan period (the late 1500s), sugar consumption was approximately one pound per person a year, but in practice, most of this sugar went to the wealthy.

Annual sugar consumption crept up to thirteen pounds per person, per year by the first part of the eighteenth century. By this time, people found they could not live without their sweet fix. Ordinary folks satisfied their cravings with low-grade sugar, as well as dried fruits and honey. Sugar loaves were given as presents to friends and offered as bribes to the influential. Only the rich could really afford to use sugar daily, but all that changed when Caribbean sugar production increased, and countries in South America began to grow sugarcane, too.

Along with these new sources of unrefined sugar came the technology to refine it. Remember, just at this time, the world was in the middle of the industrial revolution. Processors developed higher-tech refining methods similar to what we use today. Supplies were plentiful and prices plummeted, so now everybody could afford abundant, highly-refined pure sugar.

Pharmaceutical Grade Sugar

From that time, sugar evolved from a pleasant condiment to a major food item in our diet. Now, the sugar industries—including a wide variety of food processing industries and especially soft drink product industries—expend the largest advertising in the world. The average American consumes about 153 pounds of sugar a year with almost a fourth of our daily calories coming from sugar.

It shouldn't surprise us that we love sweetness. It starts when we are babies; mother's milk is very sweet. As discussed, sugar (and also honey) was relatively expensive throughout history so most desserts were not overly sweet, or not sweet at all, compared to desserts today. You can buy sugar very inexpensively now, and it is everywhere; you can't get away from it if you buy packaged foods. It is so highly-refined that it ends up as a nearly pure chemical, almost as pure as a commercial chemical or a medicine. Sugarcane contains a variety of natural minerals with balanced nutritional values, but refined sugar is a pure chemical substance of non-nutritive, empty calories that rob the body of vitamins and minerals.

Even though people began to use more sugar during the modern age (after the turn of the century and during the early 1900s), we only began to overuse it when manufacturers and marketers began to promote packaged foods in the 1950s. At the same time, manufacturers and marketers, playing on our national troubles with overweight, began to push artificial sweeteners as well. These two developments changed the American sweet tooth forever.

Dulling Our Sensitivity to Sweetness

Artificial sweeteners taste hundreds of times sweeter than sugar, and they are so inexpensive to produce. What happens

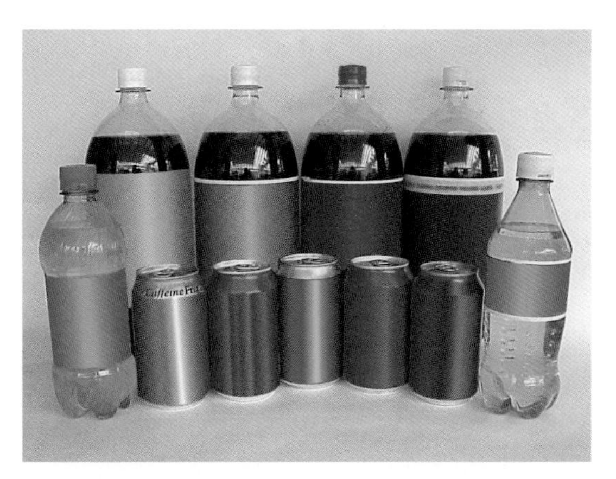

They all taste similar with little difference and excessively sweet.

when we get accustomed to very sweet stuff? We need more and more. Normally a person might be satisfied with a teaspoonful of sugar in a cup of coffee, but since most commercial foods contain sugar—and beverages and desserts contain a lot—we have become accustomed to extra sweetness. This has a direct physical effect on our taste buds. Extra sweetness—and spiciness and saltiness, too—can dull our sense of taste. It happens with our taste buds just like it does with our ear drums: loud noises over prolonged periods of time can cause hearing loss; and excessively sweet and spicy food over long periods of time can decrease taste bud sensitivity. With desensitized taste buds, we may find ourselves overeating in order to feel satisfied.

A recent study revealed that when we are overweight, we have less density of taste bud cells—or in other words, a less sensitive tongue—than we have when we are slender. For the study, volunteers were asked to taste strips of papers slightly seasoned with various flavors. The results of the research concluded that slim people could taste more of the flavors than obese individuals. Many of the seasoned papers were actually tasteless to the overweight testers, while people of normal weight could taste them.

Soft drinks are a perfect example of how this works. A sugar-sweetened soft drink contains about twelve teaspoons of pure sugar, as much as they can put in without the sugar crystallizing out, the maximum sweetness possible at drinking temperature. Diet drinks can be made even *sweeter* with chemicals. Since advertisers assure us that diet sodas have no calories, we drink them in large quantities. But if we take in that much sweetness, our taste buds grow dull, so then progressively, food needs to taste sweeter to taste good.

Providing sweet products doesn't cost the manufacturers much since both sugar and artificial sweeteners are inexpensive and easy to produce. We, the consumers, end up overdosed with both artificial sweeteners and sugar, which in large amounts are harmful to our health.

Artificial Sweeteners

Artificial sweeteners are even worse than sugar, health-wise. The most popular table sweetener, saccharine, is officially

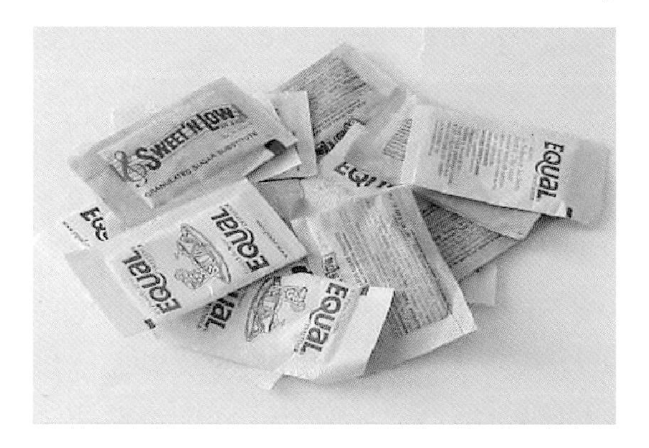

Exposed to temperatures above 86 degrees Fahrenheit, aspartame begins to break down into many toxins.

listed as an 'anticipated carcinogen.' Every package states, "Use of this product may be hazardous to your health. This product contains saccharin which has been determined to cause cancer in laboratory animals." Saccharin has a good shelf life, important for ingredients in soft drinks, and can be heated without changing the flavor. However, a chemical that stable is also hard to digest. Best of all for the processed food marketers, saccharin can be produced inexpensively. It is still widely used even though people commonly know it may cause cancer.

A newer product, aspartame, used in Nutrisweet and Equal, may be even worse. Exposed to temperatures above 86 degrees Fahrenheit, aspartame begins to break down into many toxins. Our body temperature is 98 degrees Fahrenheit, so aspartame breaks down as soon as you swallow it. Of all the toxic chemicals in aspartame, methanol is probably one of the most dangerous. When it reaches the small intestine, methanol encounters an enzyme produced by the liver which breaks it down into formaldehyde, which has been proven to cause cancer and other health problems.

As it turns out, current research has revealed that artificial sweeteners do not help us lose weight after all. Instead, they cause the body to react the same way it does with other sweeteners, by secreting insulin. This is called an *insulin reaction*, and recent studies prove that many individuals have an insulin reaction to artificial sweeteners, especially diabetics and hypoglycemics. This is relatively new information because over the years, the experts have reassured us otherwise, and most of us would never associate our obesity problems with artificial sweeteners.

Don't Throw the Baby Out with the Bath Water

After reading this, we may decide to swear off sweets altogether, but I don't think that is necessary; there's nothing inherently wrong with sugar. In fact, all foods contain some degree of sweetness; sugars in the body sustain our life. The problem comes when we overuse and abuse sweet products.

Personally, I would feel depressed if I could never again eat something sweet. Still, it's true that highly-refined sugar is problematic because in that form, sugar becomes a refined pure chemical,

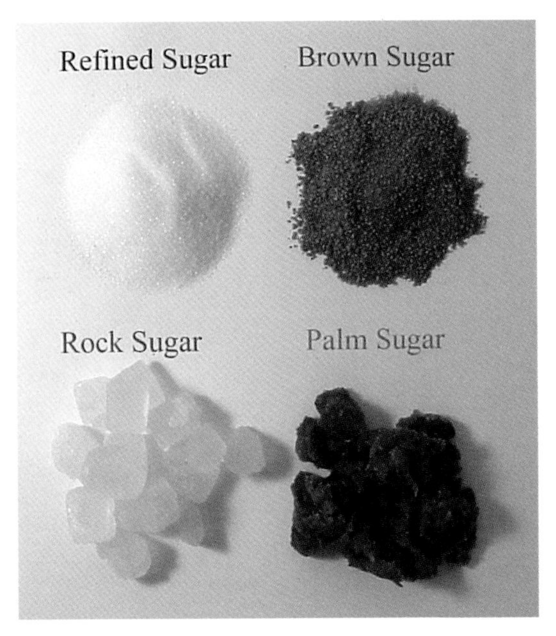

and an overdose can be toxic. An overdose of most chemicals, including salt, can be toxic as well.

What is a good approach to sugar, then? First of all, knowing that commercial products are too sweet, we might try to eat and drink less sweet stuff or dilute it to less sweetness whenever possible. Bake at home more often, use much less sugar than the recipe calls for, and consider substituting natural sweeteners, such as honey or pure maple syrup, on occasion. Less-refined sugars are available in many markets, for example, rock sugar, palm sugar, or brown sugars.

You can also buy 'raw' sugar in many supermarkets. Less-refined natural sugar is not as concentrated as pure refined sugar, and when you first see it, it may look unprocessed, even primitive, and certainly not as convenient to use. These sugars are not as sweet as refined sugar, but they contain other elements to balance the sweetness as nature intended.

My Sweet Experience

When I grew up as a boy in Taiwan, on our simple economy, we couldn't afford to buy candy or sweets at the store. Instead, we would buy sugarcane; Taiwan has the ideal climate to grow it. Sugarcane grows like bamboo in sections with a hard knot in between. There are several different varieties. We kids liked the one with brown skin, large sections, and soft texture, which was easy to chew.

In our village there were a few sugarcane stands where our pocket money could buy us a piece of cane about two feet long. The growers peeled off the skin and washed the sugarcane, and then we kids would bite off pieces, chew them, and spit out the pulp. Sugarcane juice is sweet, but not much sweeter than a ripe watermelon or a peach. It definitely isn't as sweet as a soft drink today.

For home use, we'd crush the sugarcane and squeeze it for the juice. Then we boiled off the excess water and ended up with something like candy. It was very inexpensive. As a young boy craving sweets, I had sugarcane almost everyday. It doesn't really taste like sugar; it is much less sweet, but it contains all the nutrients available in the sugarcane plant as nature provides, so I consider it to be a healthy food. A glass of ice-cold sugarcane drink is a good thirst quencher in the summertime.

If anyone got caught stealing sugarcane from one of the fields in our village, by custom, he had to pay for an opera to come and entertain the whole village. Most of us enjoyed sugarcane, yet there wasn't one fat child in our whole population, and most of us had very good health. When I finally visited a dentist in high school, I had just a few cavities, even though we had no dental care growing up and brushed our teeth with ground oyster shells or salt.

The Granddaddy of Soft Drinks

The sketches on this page, also from the *Formosa Vignette*, illustrate what people enjoyed before commercialized soft drinks. On a recent visit in Sicily, we bought fresh coconut juice from stands similar to this, and the fresh, cool coconut juice was fantastic.

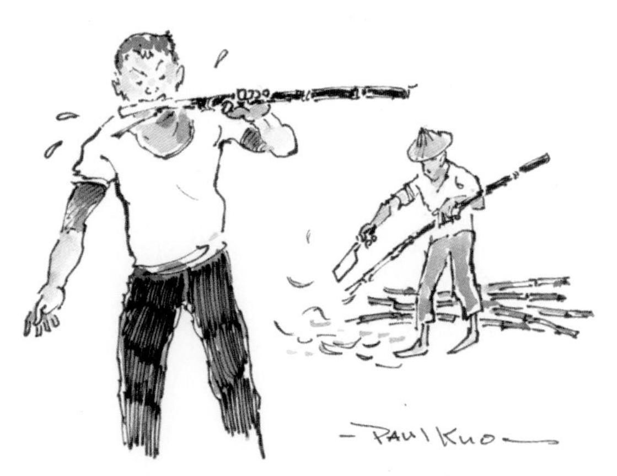

Sweet jawbreaker: "Chewing real sugarcane strengthens the jaws, cleans the molars, and maybe breaks the front teeth. You spit out the pulp, swallow the mildly sweet juice, and bite off another hunk. You may have three more feet to go."

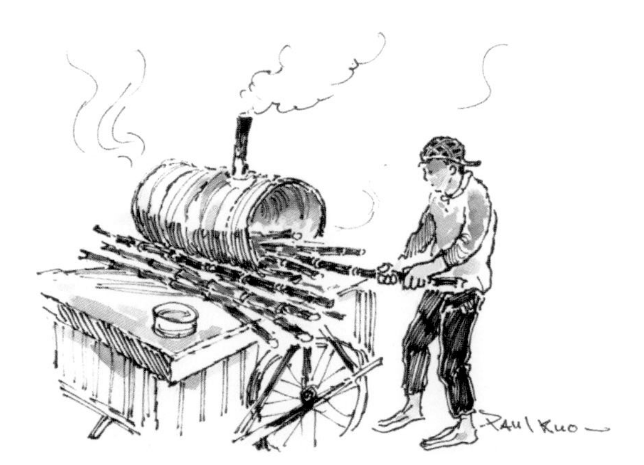

Heated sugar cane: "In order to really enjoy chewing sugarcane, you need cast-iron chewers. Some people with tender gums complained that the cold cane hurt their teeth. Hence, a new variation on an old theme, the preheated sugarcane."

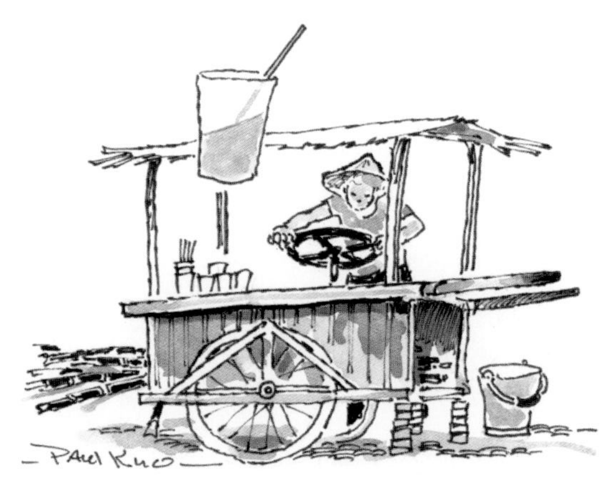

Cane espresso: "This new drink is not yet available in the PX, snack bar, or Golden Dragon Room. Walk, don't run, to the nearest street corner to get a glass of golden sugarcane juice, pressed while you wait."

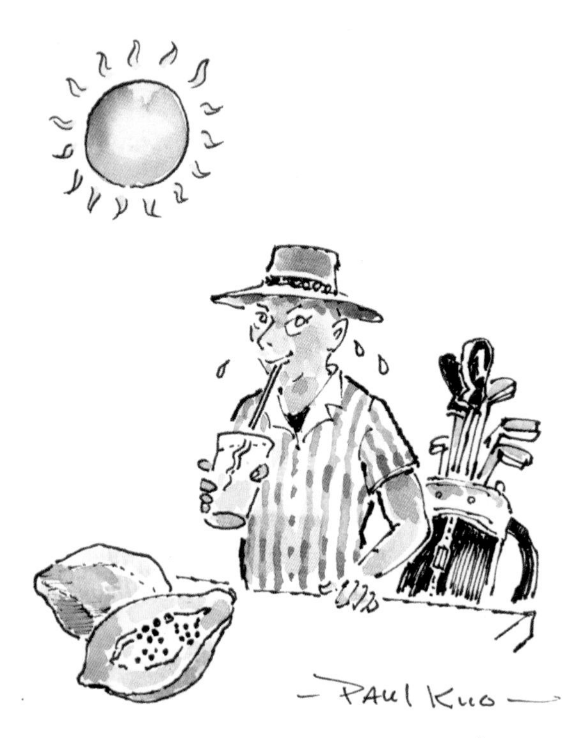

Tropical heat-aid: "The heat is here to stay, so try this in your Waring blender. The Papaya Cooler is an ice-cold melon liquefied into a delicious drink. You can also add a dash of ice cream."

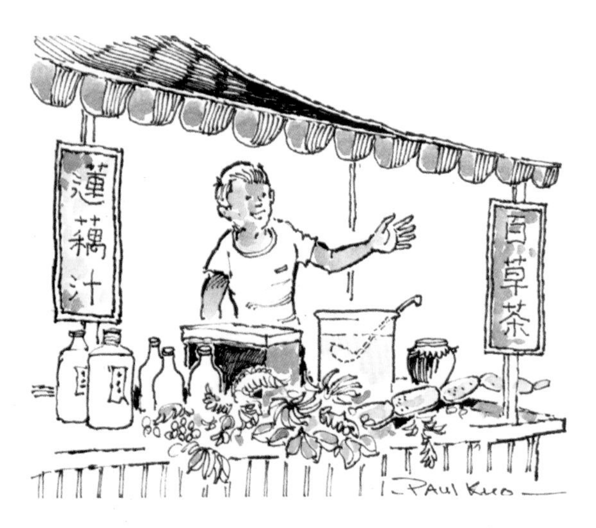

Cola grandfather: "The ancestor of all soft drinks is the Taiwan Medicinal Tea. Summertime stands offer dozens of varieties guaranteed to cool the body, refresh the soul, and ward off summer complaints. The lotus root concoction is famed for cooling you off in the summer."

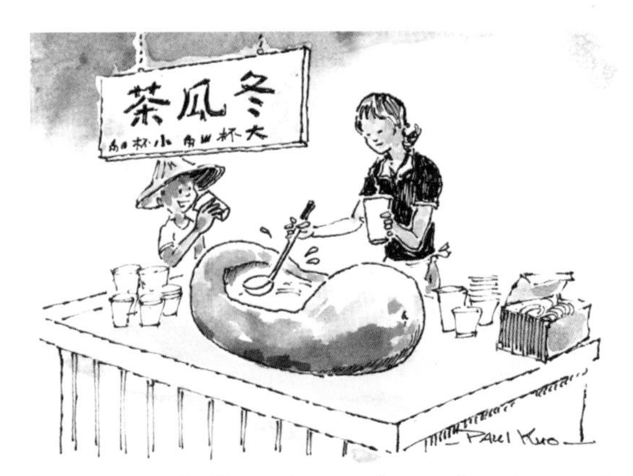

Summer squash: "This jumbo size melon is really a winter squash, a year-round favorite for delicious Chinese soup. Come summertime, this squash furnishes a well-known street-side 'kool-aid'."

Most populations around the world enjoy mild sweeteners from natural sources. When these people come to America, they often open restaurants and food stores to supply ethnic populations with foods that they are used to. For example, I often shop at ethnic bakeries—Chinese, Japanese, or Korean. The desserts there are much less sweet than American desserts. They also sell drinks made the traditional way from fruits, vegetables, or herbs. I like to buy a drink made of sugarcane and herbs to quench my summer thirst, or a preserved plum drink that has a nice fruit taste. Health food stores and popular stores such as Trader Joe's in California also stock imported bakery products and traditional drinks from other cultures. Recently at Trader Joe's, I bought French chocolate and Italian tiramisu. They were wonderful and not overpoweringly sweet.

You can also buy not-so-sweet soft drinks at these stores.

You Don't Have to Give Up Sweets

Although it may not seem like it at first, you can easily get used to a milder sweet taste. After a while, you may find that the typical American treats begin to taste too sweet. Soft drinks will seem especially oversweet, and you can taste the chemicals in them, too. I suggest that, as a rule, you don't drink soda pop much at all. It is better to drink tea or water. But this doesn't mean that you need to give up sweets entirely. Most traditional meals serve some kind of sweet food at the end of the meal, something light and mildly sweet. For example, most Chinese restaurants offer free almond Jell-O with fruit cocktail; ginger-flavored, sweet, soft bean curd; small sesame or almond cookies; and other similar desserts. If you get a dessert that is too sweet, take a smaller portion so that you will reduce your sugar intake.

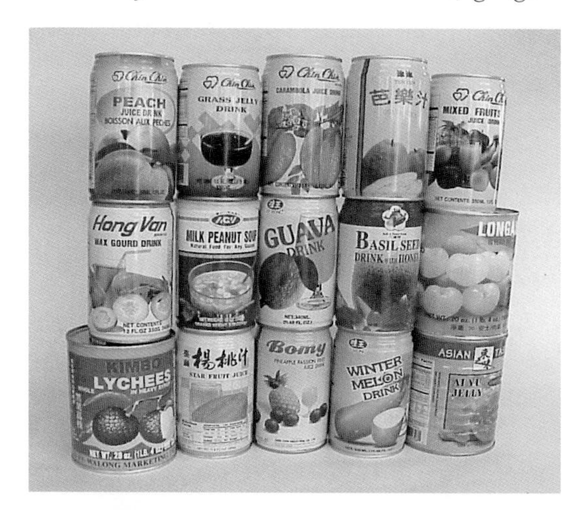

Chinese drinks. The drinks pictured are Basil Seed drink, Guava drink, Grass Jelly drink, Winter Melon drink, Passion Fruit drink, and Star Fruit drink, etc. Each has a unique, distinct, natural taste and flavor, and is sweetened (mildly) with cane sugar and honey.

When you prepare your own desserts at home, try using raw sugar or, as I mentioned above, reduce the amounts of regular sweeteners called for in the recipe. You'll be surprised how good it tastes. Have fruit and cheese for dessert occasionally, and gently wean your family from highly-sweetened desserts. Homemade desserts with less sugar will help them get used to treats that are less sweet. In fact, I have found that if you make homemade cookies, you can use much less sugar in the recipe, and then sprinkle a bit of sugar on each cookie before it goes in the oven. The initial taste of the cookie will be quite sweet even though there's not that much sugar in the recipe.

Like many traditional populations around the world, you may soon find that you really enjoy less sweet foods. It's a good way to improve your health and help lose weight, too.

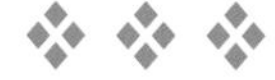

PART THREE

Food for Thought: Better for Us

Once we understand what we're really doing with our diet, we can begin to improve the way we eat. Despite popular trends today, carbohydrates remain an important part of a healthy diet, and most of us depend on bread. We buy our bread readymade from the market and eat it over several days. Old bread takes more liquid to wash down, so we use plenty of soda pop for that. Part Three endeavors to offer alternatives and paves the way toward helping you modify and improve your diet.

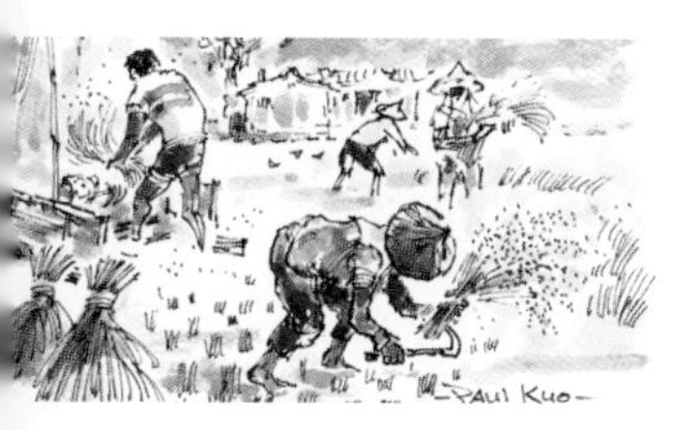

In **Chapter Seven** we focus on rice. This staple food for many populations around the world is often perceived by Americans as too difficult and cumbersome to prepare, especially for our busy modern life. This chapter shows you how to prepare delicious rice dishes effortlessly.

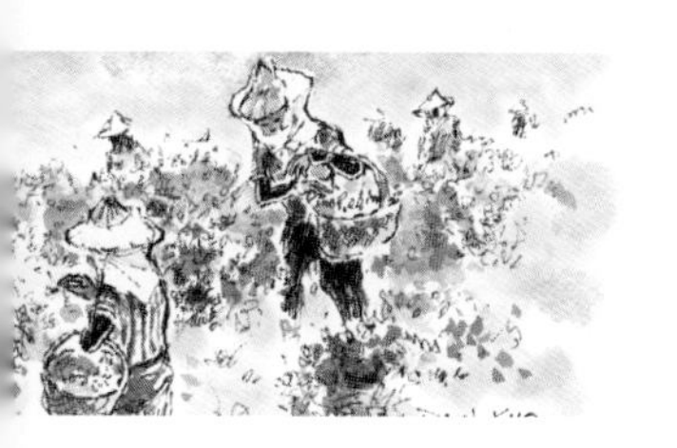

Chapter Eight provides everything you need to know about tea and how to make it a healthy and delicious alternative for your mealtime beverages. I encourage you to drink more tea with meals for good health. After reading this chapter about tea, you will be surprised to find out how much you don't know about tea.

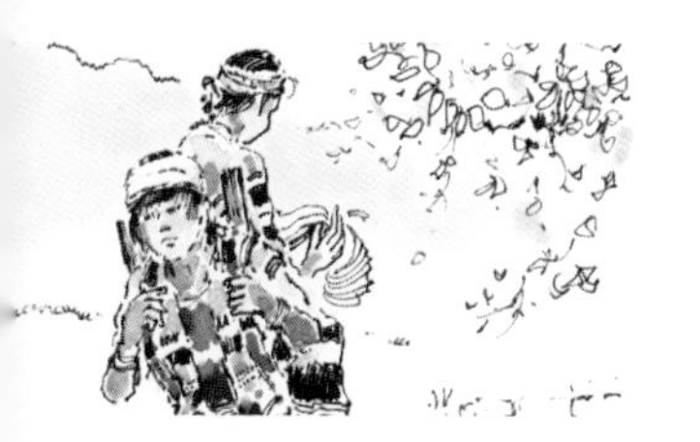

In **Chapter Nine** we familiarize you with some basic items regarding herbs and spices. Herbs and spices have been used in cooking by our ancestors for eons. They enhance the flavor of the dishes, and most of these ingredients contain important nutrients. The basic cooking techniques covered in this chapter provide a foundation for those discussed in the subsequent chapters.

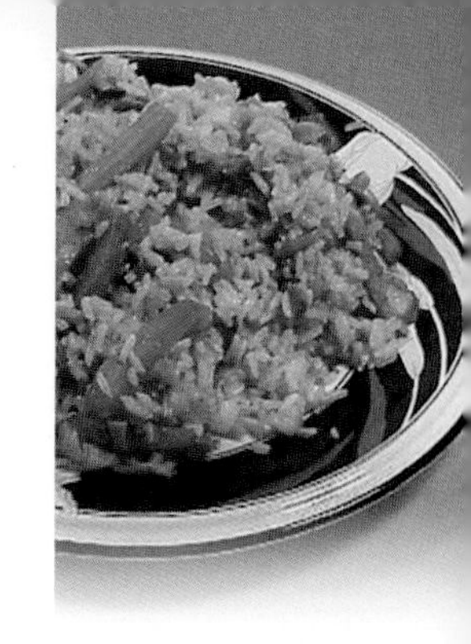

Chapter 7
Staple Foods: Rice

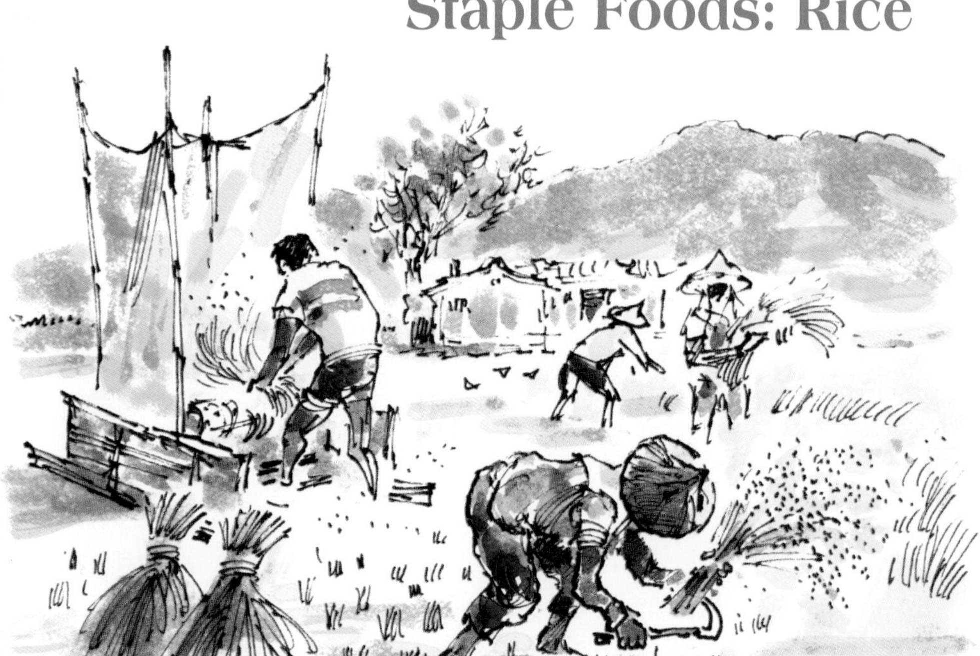

Traditionally, for their staple foods, most ethnic groups eat carbohydrates (or starches) from plants that were originally common weeds or grasses. These plants are easy to grow and produce plenty of seeds or roots, which provide an abundance of nutrients. Carbohydrates provide the basic fuel we need for energy, as well as many other nutrients we need to keep our complex body systems healthy.

The most common starches are wheat, rice, potatoes, and corn, though wheat and rice are probably the most common carbohydrates eaten today. Wheat and rice are seeds that mature in spikelets, which serve the same function as eggshells: the outer coating provides protection that allows the seed to germinate. We eat the seeds themselves, and in times of a good harvest, we feed animals our grain surplus to produce meat.

Rice Varieties

The rice we have today originates from a family of wild grass and comes in hundreds of varieties, though only a selected few varieties are cultivated for popular consumption. Different areas in the world grow their own particular varieties of rice, all with various names and flavors. *Arborio* is the rice preferred by Italians for risotto while the Japanese and Taiwanese prefer the waxy or glutenous, slightly sticky, medium-grain variety known in this country as *Cal Rose*.

There are about twenty varieties of rice grown commercially in the United States. Today, six states produce more than 99 percent of all the rice grown in America: Arkansas, California, Louisiana, Mississippi, Missouri, and Texas. Arkansas is the largest rice producing state in the nation—about 45 percent of total production in America. The medium grain variety known as Cal Rose is produced in California, while long grain and others are produced in the other five states. The Japanese and Taiwanese prefer Cal Rose. Popular sushi rice is Cal Rose. Jasmine rice, a long grain variety, has a distinct aroma favored by Chinese and other populations in Southeast Asia. In America, many people prefer the long grain rice grown in the southern states. As I mentioned, Cal Rose is a little sticky when cooked; most of the different types of rice are the non-sticky variety. The stickiness of a variety of rice is determined by the amount of water-soluble amylase starch in the inner kernels of the rice. The less amylase starch, the stickier the rice.

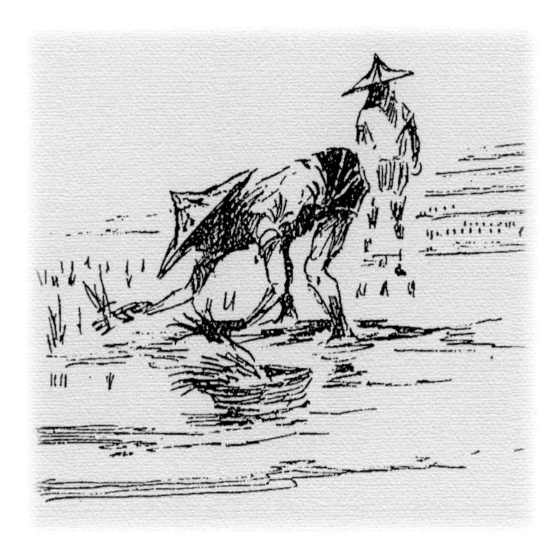

Fertile Taiwan. Two crops of rice a year is common in most parts of Taiwan. Here the rice seedlings are planted in the wet paddy. It's a back breaking job, but Taiwan's rice bowl must be filled.

Brown Rice. The rice kernel is encased in a coat called bran and surrounded by a tough fibrous hull. Brown rice is the kernel with the hull removed; it contains bran and the embryo, or germ. Many

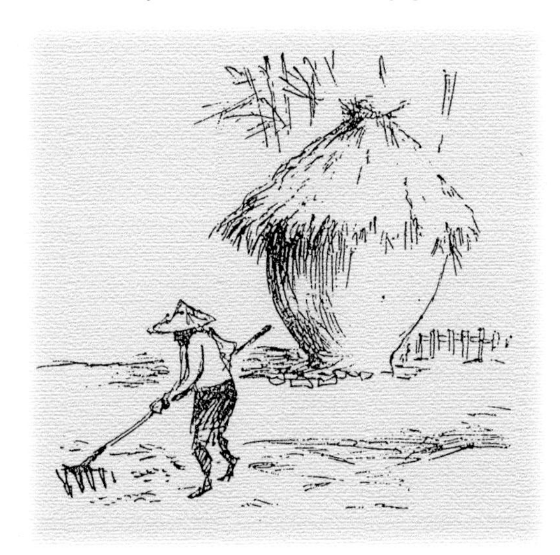

Rice bin. A picturesque part of Central and Southern Taiwan scenery is this rice bin. A huge wicker basket is first made and then covered with clay. Topped with a grass roof, it serves as an inexpensive storage place for grain.

people mistakenly think brown rice is a kind of brown-colored rice. Brown rice comes in many different colors depending on the variety. Pay a visit to a well-stocked natural food store, gourmet specialty shop, or health food store and you will find rice from Himalayan red, Chinese black, to Purple Thai and every color in between.

Wild Rice. Wild rice is naturally abundant in the cold rivers and lakes of Minnesota and Canada; wild rice was the staple in the diet of the Chippewa and Sioux Indians native to this region. It has a mixture of colors. These varieties of rice are for special occasions and are not consumed regularly.

Parboiled Rice. When the brown rice is polished, the bran and germ are removed and it becomes white rice, which most people prefer. Unfortunately, most of the valuable minerals and vitamins are lost in the polishing process. The perfect solution to good-tasting and nutritious rice is to use converted or parboiled rice. With converted rice, the whole grain of rice is steamed before milling, which drives the valuable nutrients found in the germ and bran into the heart of the kernel. Thus, the converted rice has a nutritional content higher than white rice and a bit lower than brown rice. The only problem is that converted rice is more expensive; it is a value-added product.

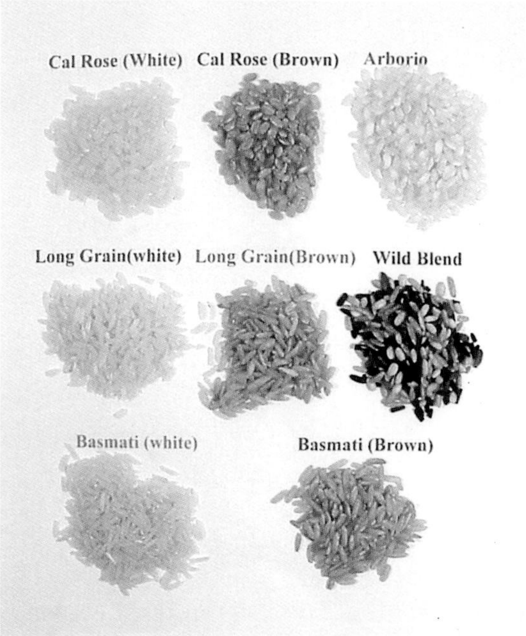

Bread Versus Rice

Wheat bread has been our staple food ever since our forefathers brought it over from the Old World. We would all agree that a piece of fresh-baked bread makes our mouth water and is one of the most enjoyable parts of the meal. However, with our modern lifestyle, almost none of us can eat fresh bread every day. Most of us shop once or twice a week, and the commercial bread we buy is mass-produced in factories, so it contains many chemicals to keep it looking good and fresh for a long period of time. Fresh home-baked bread is great but not practical for our lifestyles since most of us don't bake at home and don't make daily trips to the store. Day-old and older bread does not taste as good, but we have learned to live with it.

In addition, in recent years, wheat allergies have become very common. Many people can't eat wheat products because they cause a powerful glucose reaction, dangerous for diabetics and problematic for the overweight since a glucose reaction stimulates weight gain. It is well known that rice is easier for our body to digest than wheat; therefore, rice is a great alternative.

Automatic Rice Cookers

Unfortunately, many people think that rice is difficult to cook, but nothing could be easier. The best solution is an automatic rice cooker. These rice cookers have been standard kitchenware in almost all Asian families since the 1960s. It is a shame most Americans don't know how useful they are. Most Americans are still boiling or microwaving rice. You can buy automatic rice cookers in most department stores. Any Asian market will have them as well. Prices range from $25 to perhaps $200.

You may be surprised at how easy it is to use your rice cooker. You just put pre-measured rice and water inside the pot, and when the rice is cooked and the water has absorbed or evaporated, the temperature rises and the cooker automatically switches

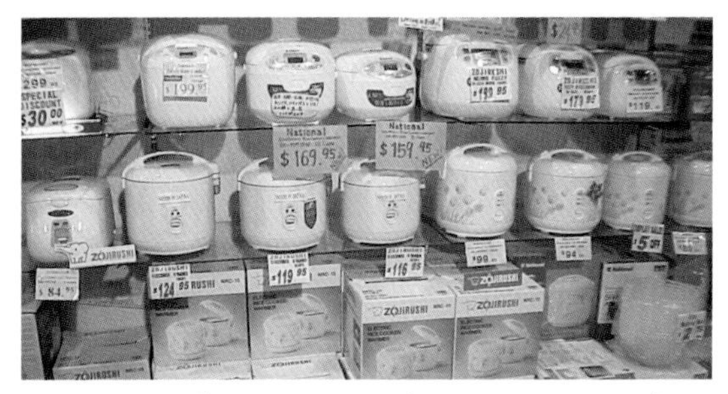

An assortment of automatic rice cookers in a Japanese market.

from 'cook' mode to 'warm' mode to keep the rice warm for serving. It takes only twenty minutes to automatically cook rice.

You can use your rice cooker for other things as well, such as steaming vegetables and other foods. One of my friends found it superb for steaming tamales. Every rice cooker comes with an instruction booklet that shows you how to use it. There are even expensive models that can keep the rice warm and ready to eat for days. Personally, I prefer the regular models since I can make fresh rice for every meal easily and inexpensively. Rice cookers come in various sizes so you can buy one that is appropriate for your family.

With your automatic rice cooker, it is impossible to make a mistake cooking rice. In the old days, cooking rice with a wood-burning stove required great skill and care. Most of the time, the rice overcooked and burned the bottom of the pot. Overcooked rice sticks to the bottom of the pot, and it happened almost every time on wood stoves. To avoid the waste of throwing away the burned rice, Oriental cooks invented pot-sticker soup, which was made by pouring water into the pot to remove the rice stuck to the bottom. After boiling, the water took on a nice flavor and, with the addition of vegetables and meat, cooks developed a tasty soup dish. Today, in many Chinese and Persian restaurants, pot sticker rice is very popular. The main ingredient, burned rice, is processed for commercial use since with modern rice cookers, you cannot make pot-sticker rice even if you try.

A nice benefit of eating rice is how inexpensive it is. Daily rice costs *much* less than daily bread. In America, you can buy rice almost everywhere, and in big cities, you can buy rice from around the globe. In fact, we have the best selection of varieties from all over the world here in the U.S. We produce ample supplies of domestic rice and, consequently, we have the lowest rice prices in the world. Most of the time you can buy rice in bulk, in bags weighing between five to fifty pounds.

It is easy and more economical to buy the bulk rice, store it in a large plastic container, and have it readily available. Cooking it in your automatic rice cooker will give you an inexpensive, almost-instant staple food whenever you need it.

Brown Rice for Your Health

As with bread, white rice or polished rice is most popular, and almost all restaurants and most households serve white rice. The brown rice, which retains the bran and germ, is indisputably the best grain for our health. It is rich in vitamins and minerals and has lots of fiber. But brown rice, like whole-grain wheat, can be rough and dry tasting. Fortunately, there are ways to prepare brown rice that are both delicious and nutritious. For softer rice like Cal Rose, adding extra water is enough to cook the rice tender and give it a nice texture. It takes about three parts water to one part of brown rice, while with regular rice, the ratio is two to one.

Some varieties of brown rice can have a very hard outer layer and need more than just extra cooking water. For these, you can soak the brown rice in water prior to cooking. Place the water and rice in the refrigerator for about a day, or overnight, and then cook the rice the

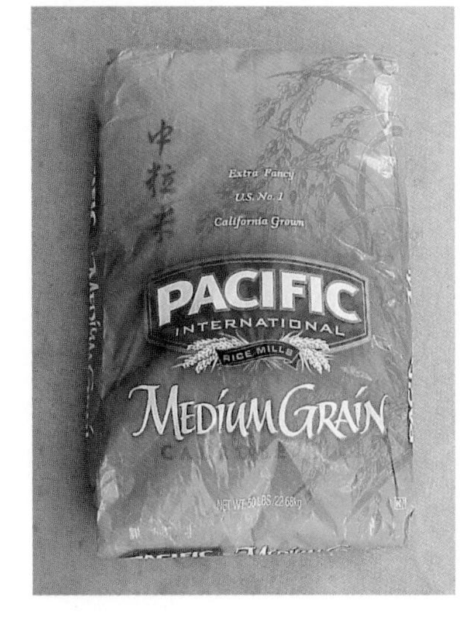

regular way in the rice cooker with extra water. How long you soak the rice, and the amount of cooking water determines the tenderness of the finished rice. Soak it at least overnight, although some rice may take twenty-four hours.

Be sure to refrigerate the rice when you soak it, or it can start to go bad. Brown rice boils over more easily and can make a mess on the counter top, so keep an eye on it. You can cook a week's supply, save part of it in the freezer, and then place a couple of days' supply in the refrigerator. Just reheat the rice to serve it using a microwave, steamer, or frying pan. Cooked rice dries out easily; therefore, to reheat it, add a small amount of water for moist rice.

Various Ways to Eat Rice

If you like soft, tender rice, California medium-grain, brown rice is the best choice; it is available in most Asian markets and at many warehouse grocery stores.

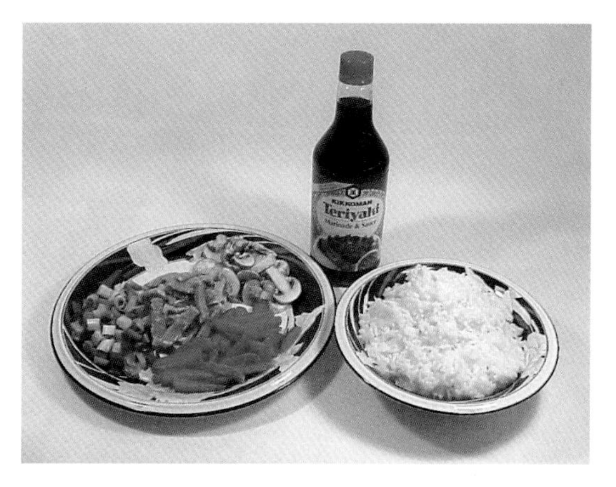

Brown rice tastes particularly good made into fried rice. Simple fried rice can be made with just green onions, bacon or ham, and soy sauce. First, cut about one stalk of green onion per bowl of rice into one quarter to three eighths inch pieces. Cut bacon or ham into about three eighths to one half inch pieces. It is good to add vegetables such as carrots, mushrooms, peas, or corn.

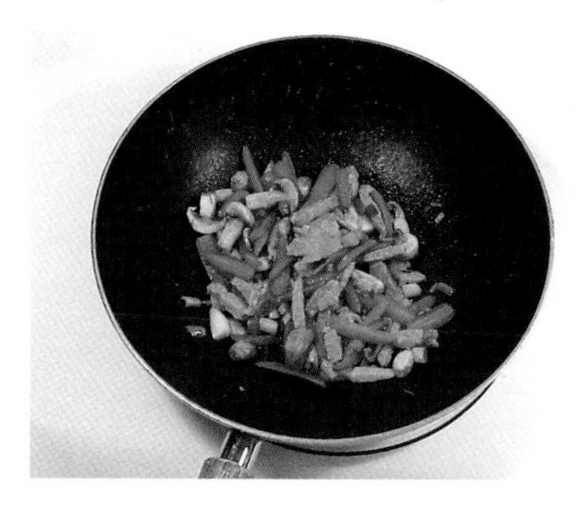

Place about one tablespoon of olive oil per bowl of rice into a hot frying pan. Place both the cut green onion and the bacon or ham into the pan and sauté a few seconds until the bacon is cooked.

Place cooked rice into the pan and stir it with a chopstick or spatula. Season with soy sauce or teriyaki sauce, then add a couple tablespoonfuls of water or soup stock to make the rice more moist. Stir it to make sure it's mixed properly. Bacon and ham are salty, so be careful and go easy with the soy sauce and salt.

Fried rice can be saved in the fridge for about five days, or up to six months

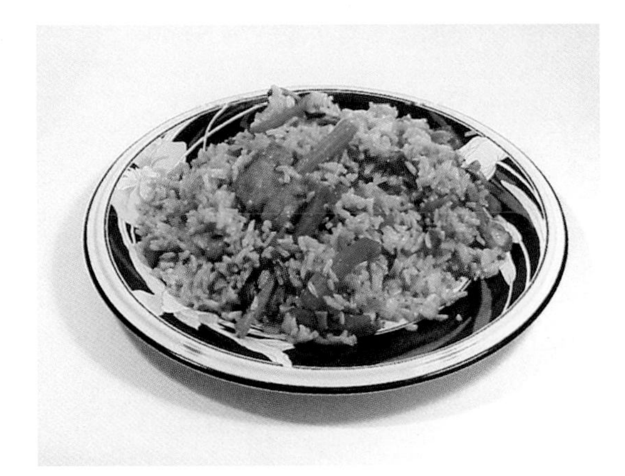

in the freezer; just add water to reheat it, the same as regular cooked rice. You can make up a week's supply of fried rice over the weekend and refrigerate it for use during the week.

You might like to try a Taiwanese method of cooking rice. Add one-inch cubes of peeled yams, potatoes, or sweet potatoes to cook together with the rice. This alters the aroma and taste of the rice slightly and adds nutritional value and a smooth texture. You can also add legumes such as beans to the rice to create a different meal every time with even higher nutritional values.

To get started, look in the supermarket for a package with a mixture of grains, usually five different grains. As for the beans, soybeans have the highest food values and health properties. Fresh precooked and peeled, green frozen soybeans can be added just as the rice finishes cooking.

The rice cooker can improve your diet dramatically if you'll give it a chance. You can get the rice ready in the morning and set a preset timer on the rice cooker, and the steaming rice will be ready when it's time to put dinner together. Doing this, you'll be halfway finished making dinner before you even get home. Once you adopt this routine, you'll find that it provides more time to make creative and nutritious hot meals at home—so you can avoid the junk-food temptation at dinnertime.

Keep in mind that you can use the same basic technique discussed here and replace rice with noodles for variety. Vegetarians can use soy protein substitutes such as imitation bacon or even seasoned, firm tofu instead of bacon and come up with an equally delicious and nutritious dish.

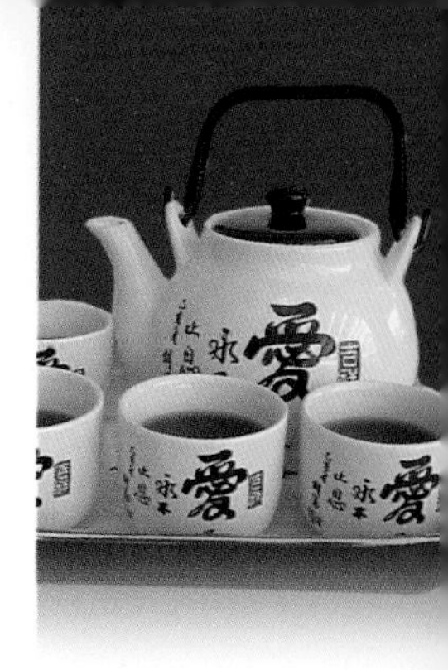

Chapter 8
Tea

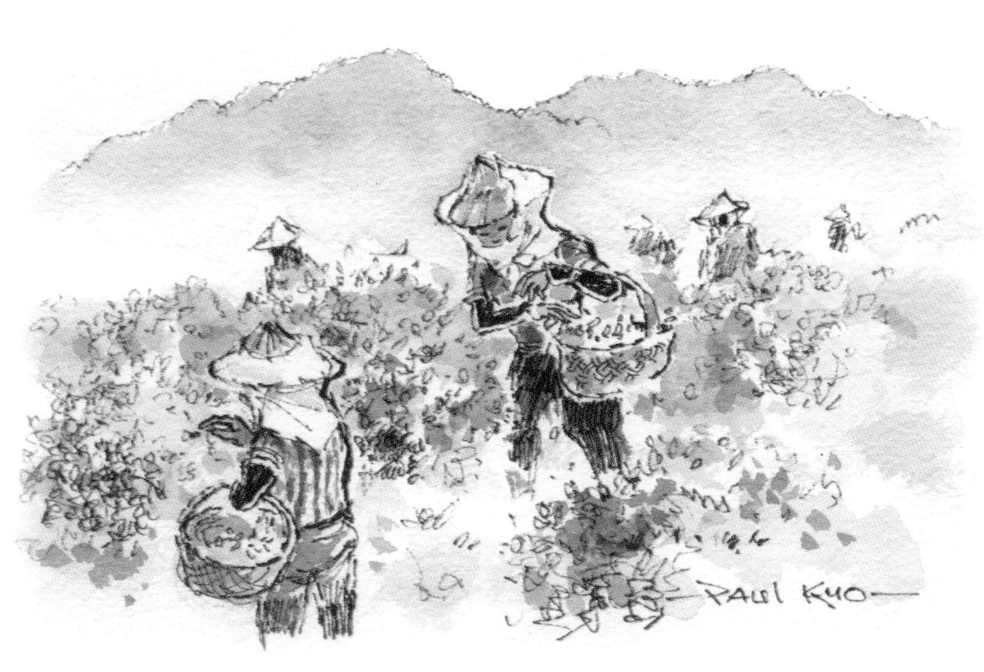

Drinking liquids has always been a very important part of human culture—to wash down foods, quench thirst, and warm ourselves—and as a pleasant social custom. As mentioned many times, soft drinks are harmful to our health because they contain so much sugar (or worse, artificial sweeteners) and chemicals. Natural drinks such as water, juice, milk, coffee, and tea are better choices. Just about everybody drinks coffee and tea, and people sometimes equate coffee with tea, but they are very different substances. We all know coffee comes from the seeds or beans of coffee trees, while tea comes from the leaves of tea plants. They have nothing in common except they both make good beverages. Tea has always been popular in the Orient and in the British Isles and is becoming more and more popular in America as well.

A Brief History of Tea

Based on Chinese legend, a famous experimental herbalist, Shen Nong, who was researching medicinal plants, discovered tea accidentally in China about 3000 B.C. According to the legend, one day the leaves of the tea plant fell into water he was boiling outdoors. He tasted the resulting drink and liked it; he also found that it was a good antidote for poisoning, something he evidently needed in his plant-tasting experiments.

Tea has been a most important part of life in Asia for thousands of years. The first tea reached Europe around 1610 on Dutch ships. By the end of the seventeenth century, tea had become popular in Dutch and British high society, and American colonists brought it to the New World.

On December 16, 1773, the Boston Tea Party, which involved the destruction of a shipload of tea, protested the high taxes on imported tea, which contributed to the general unrest and ultimate birth of this nation. It shows how highly valued tea was, both to the Colonists and to England.

Health Benefits of Tea

For thousands of years, tea has been known to be beneficial to health. In my youth, first thing in the morning, my mother would make tea for my grandmother. It was believed to clear the throat, relieve congestion in the chest, stimulate saliva, emulsify fat, help digestion, and have an overall cleansing effect on the body. Tea was served to Grandma on bitter, cold, winter days as well as hot summer days; in fact, it was served all year round, and she was given more when she had a cold.

In recent years, scientists all over the world have been studying tea for its medicinal value. According to the studies, tea is packed with antioxidant compounds twenty times as powerful as vitamin E and 200 times as powerful as vitamin C. So far, three health-promoting components of tea have been identified: caffeine, polyphenols (groups of strong antioxidant chemical substances), and aromatic essential oils. As you learn more about some of the results of tea research in the following paragraphs, you may want to drink more tea.

Tea May Inhibit Cancer. The strong antioxidative action of polyphenols inhibits mutation of DNA in healthy cells. These mutations can cause cells to become cancerous. Teas may also inhibit or block the action of cancer-causing substances. Reports have indicated that the stomach cancer rate has been remarkably low in the tea-growing district of Shizuoka, Japan, Sichuan, and Jiangsu provinces in China. Scientists concluded that in these tea-growing areas, people drank tea often and drank it strong. In areas with a higher stomach cancer mortality, people favored weak tea and drank it infrequently. Studies have shown that antioxidants made from tea, applied to the skin, significantly inhibited growth of induced skin cancer in mice.

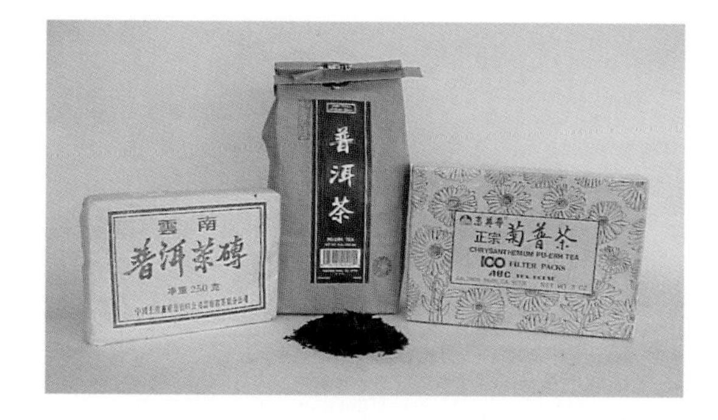

Tea May Help Your Heart. Traditionally, tea has been known as a mild circulatory stimulant. Research has shown that tea strengthens blood vessels, reduces absorption of cholesterol in the gut, and decreases the blood's tendency to form clots. A University of California survey found a reduction in atherosclerosis in tea drinkers as compared to coffee drinkers. In tests, animals fed a high fat diet *and tea* had less severe sclerotic lesions in the aorta than a control group that did not receive the tea.

Tea May Also Have a Slimming Effect. There is a special tea available, on request, in many authentic Chinese restaurants called *Pu-Erh* tea. It has an 'old and earthy' aroma, and a strong, dark tea color, but a mild taste. It is commonly believed that this tea reduces fat in the bloodstream and in the tissues. It is famed for its medicinal properties, specifically for relief from indigestion and diarrhea. This tea is a broadleafed tea tree growing in Yuennan Province in a mountainous area near the Tibetan border. Recent studies indicate Pu-Erh tea is effective in reducing cholesterol, triglycerides, and body weight. It received the Ninth International Food Award at a conference in Barcelona, Spain, in 1986. In a meal with lots of fat, such as a *dim sum* tea lunch, Pu-Erh tea is frequently consumed to combat the fat in the meal.

There are diet teas on the market as well, which are mostly a mixture of oolong tea and other ingredients. But why worry about tea as a diet drink or a medicine? Let's just treat tea as a good beverage, one of life's enjoyments that just happens to be extremely good for us.

Tea May Help You Live Longer. The Chinese have always believed that tea drinking promotes longevity. In recent Chinese studies, they discovered that fruit flies given tea had more than double the average life spans, from an average 16.5 to 40.5 days, compared to a control group of flies that were not fed tea.

Tea May Kill Germs. Numerous studies have shown that tea has germicidal properties as well. It has also been shown to substantially reduce the growth of oral bacteria, reducing cavities.

Considering the negative side effects of soda pop and other popular beverages, tea begins to look like a very good choice indeed. However, don't be fooled by the canned or bottled teas like Snapple and

Arizona tea. Read the ingredients. Most of these teas are just like soda pop, full of sugar, artificial sweeteners, chemicals, and artificial flavors. The research shows again and again the health benefits of natural tea, which make it an ideal choice for our everyday beverage. But to reap these benefits, it is best to make your own.

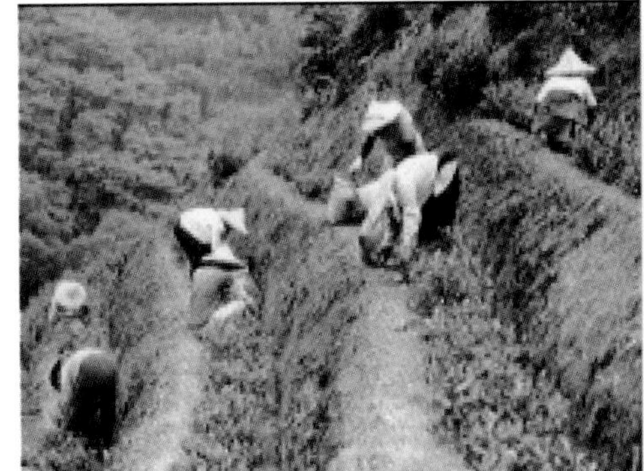
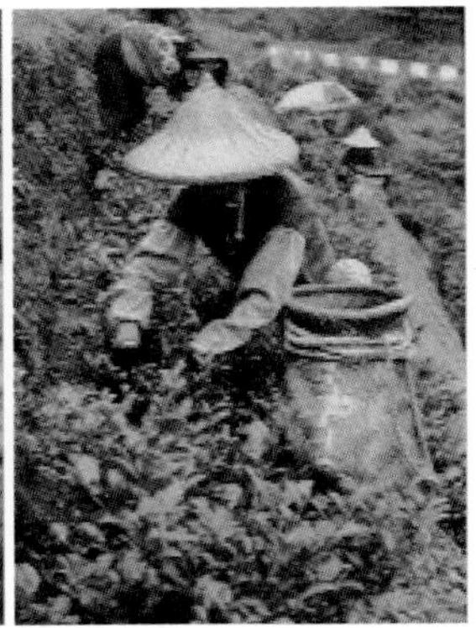
Hand-picked harvesting for good quality tea at a typical terraced tea plantation in Taiwan.

Not All 'Teas' Are Created Equal

Recently, marketers are taking advantage of the health hype about tea by introducing numerous 'tea' drinks on the market. Of course, not all teas are the same. Of the teas that are marketed, only those made from the leaves of the plant *Camellia sinensis* (sinensis is Latin for Chinese) have revealed the previously mentioned health benefits. The 'herbal teas' should not be confused with real tea. It may not be a surprise to you that the tea we drink in America, and the way we drink it, is very different from the way tea is consumed in Asia.

What Is Tea?

Tea is made from the leaves of the tea plant, and there are many varieties of tea plants. Various strains, differences in topography, soil, and climate in diverse growing areas, and methods of processing all combine to create different types of tea. Good tea plants grow at high elevations.

Just as there are three general types of wines—white wine, red wine, and rosé (in between)—there are three different types of teas; green tea, oolong tea, and black tea, which the Chinese call red tea. In principle, processing the leaves in different ways creates different teas even when the same variety of tea plant is used. In practice, certain strains, localities, and climatic conditions, etc., determine the optimum types of teas that can be produced in any particular area. For example, black tea is fermented; oolong is semi-fermented; and green tea is not fermented at all—and they all start with the same tea plant. Because green tea is not fermented, it may retain delicate, multiple, complex chemicals, which may be destroyed or altered during fermentation.

Not surprisingly, certain varieties grown in particular areas make the best tea.

Quality of Tea

I have enjoyed my share of wining and dining in many business and social settings. Often the most expensive, rare wines that everyone seems to enjoy will not taste good to me, while inexpensive wines with a simple, basic flavor taste good. The same goes for tea. People often have a distinct preference for certain kinds. Nevertheless, here are some criteria for good quality tea. The best tea comes from the early spring harvest while the leaves are young and tender, and therefore, more flavorful.

During a visit to a famous tea-growing area in Taiwan, I was told that the time of day and position of the moon during harvest affected the quality of the tea. The choice parts to pick are 'one or two leaves and a bud.' The fine hair on the leaf bud and underside of the leaf is believed to impart the finest flavor to the tea. Teas with incomplete leaves, and fragments of tea leaves, produce inferior quality tea. Quality tea leaves are glossy rather than dull.

As with wine, the quality of tea is judged from its aroma, appearance, taste, and after-taste. Tea is also judged by its ability to cleanse the palate and its soothing effect on the throat as you drink it. Fine tea should have a good aroma and a fresh and soothing taste. A good cup of tea should be clear and bright with light, appropriate coloring depending on the type of tea. A dull, unclear, and muddy cup of tea is always a sign of low quality.

The tea prepared for commercial tea bags is machine picked, blended, and processed to maintain brand flavor consistency, and it's priced for popular use. There's a world of difference between that tea and quality tea. Tea bags sealed in paper lose most of their essential, aromatic oils; most quality bags are sealed in aluminum foil.

Again, as with wine, high quality teas are marketed and priced according to their variety, location, processing, and year. Good quality tea such as the Taiwanese Don Ting oolong tea and the Chinese Dragon Well green tea will always be more expensive. Some teas are scented and named after the scent such as jasmine, rose, orchid, and many fruit teas. These are not herbal teas; they just have added aromatic components.

Most tea can be served any time, but like wine, some teas are better in certain circumstances. For example, just as white wine is good with seafood and red wine is better with meat, green jasmine tea is good with seafood, and strong black tea is better with heavier meats.

About Decaf Tea

Caffeine stimulates the heart and respiratory systems to bring more oxygen to the brain, thus increasing mental alertness. It is also believed to help digestion and kidney function. However, there has been much concern in the United States about the possible negative health effects of caffeine; therefore, decaf tea is available.

What is decaf tea? Caffeine can be dissolved out of tea with liquid carbon dioxide, ethyl acetate, or methylene chloride, which has been identified as a carcinogen. Among these three ways to remove caffeine, the liquid carbon dioxide method is considered the best. It produces a minimum loss of antioxidants and no toxic chemical residue, which can occur with the other two methods. The other two methods reduce antioxidants in excessive amounts; in addition, the methylene chloride residue may remain in the tea. You cannot assume that a manufacturer's claim of 'natural decaffeination' on the label is always correct, and there is no practical way to assess the method of decaffeination that was used.

Just like other processed foods, additives or chemicals can be added to improve the aroma or cosmetic appearance of teas. Tea contains less caffeine than coffee, and green tea contains the least. Rather than drinking decaf tea, it is better to take the approach of drinking less or weaker tea, or drinking mild green tea if caffeine intake is a concern.

How to Make a Cup of Tea

Usually, when we order a cup of tea, we are served with a pot of hot water and a tea bag. We just open the cover and place the bag into the pot. Some dip the tea bag a few times and remove it, while others place the bag inside the pot and pour the tea as needed. We all know that steeping the bag longer makes stronger tea. Tea bags are convenient and practical. Today, there are many varieties of expensive tea bags coming from all over the world and available in gourmet stores or coffee shops. In addition, there are many pure teas (just tea— no sweetener, fruit, or other additive) in cans next to the soda in Asian markets. And this is the sum of all we moderns know about making a cup of tea.

Tea connoisseurs do not like tea bags; they believe that it's not the real thing. The tea inside the tea bags is not made with whole tea leaves, but crumbled leaves instead. It infuses promptly, but the quality of the tea suffers. The essential oils of the tea create the aroma of the tea, and they are volatile and delicate. Unfortunately, they evaporate during handling and storage, especially if the leaves

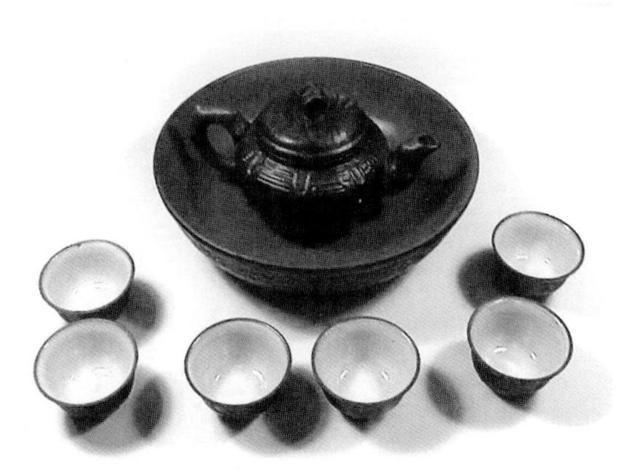

Traditional tea set

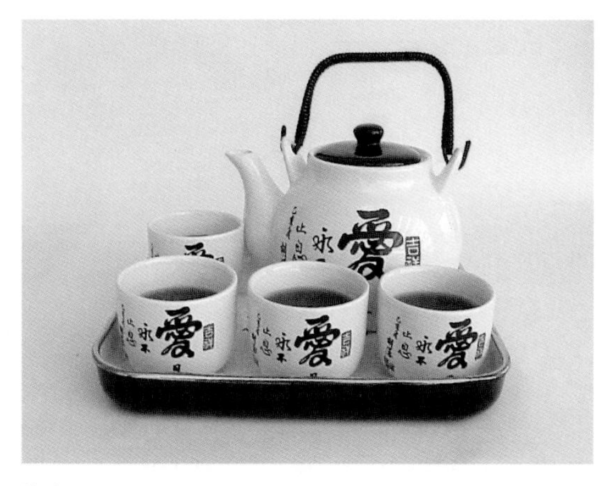

Modern tea set

are crumbled. Most Asians still insist on 'the real thing.'

So What Is Real Tea?

During a recent visit to Taiwan, I was interested to learn that the economic boom on the island and the newly discovered health benefits of tea have created a renaissance for tea drinking. On every single visit to friends and acquaintances, tea was offered to me immediately. Serving a cup of tea is a symbol of showing respect, the joy of welcome, and togetherness. For a visitor to reject a cup of tea can be considered rude.

Each household has a tea set consisting of a cart with a butane stove, a tray, a tiny teapot, and a few small cups without handles about the size of a sake cup or half of an eggshell.

Water is boiled in a large kettle. The teapot and cups are rinsed with boiling water first, and then the pot is loosely filled with tea leaves, a lot of tea for a small pot. Boiling water is poured into the pot and the water is drained immediately to rinse the tea leaves of any impurities that may harm the flavor. Finally, the pot full of leaves is filled with water and allowed to stand for a couple of minutes, and then the tea is served.

The first pour of the tea is savored for its aroma. Then the pot is filled with more boiling water and steeped for a few minutes. The second pouring of tea has the most flavor because it has reached its full strength. On the third pouring, the aroma has diminished quite a bit, but the flavor and taste are still strong.

During my visits, I was delighted that the conversation almost always turned to tea. These are a few things I learned: the perforated infuser or tea ball, which Westerners often use, prevents the water from fully saturating the leaves, and therefore, is not satisfactory. Very fine tea takes a shorter steeping time. Do not keep the pot warm with a padded cozy because it causes the leaves to be over-steeped. Don't steep too long; if you want stronger tea, use more tea leaves. Color is not a good gauge of flavor; rather, timing it properly is the most important. A cup of tea has to be clear with a reflective, slightly green or orange color depending on the variety. It should taste clean, soothe your throat, stimulate the salivary glands, and quench your thirst. If it tastes bitter or too strong and lacks aroma, it probably steeped too long or the tea leaves were too old.

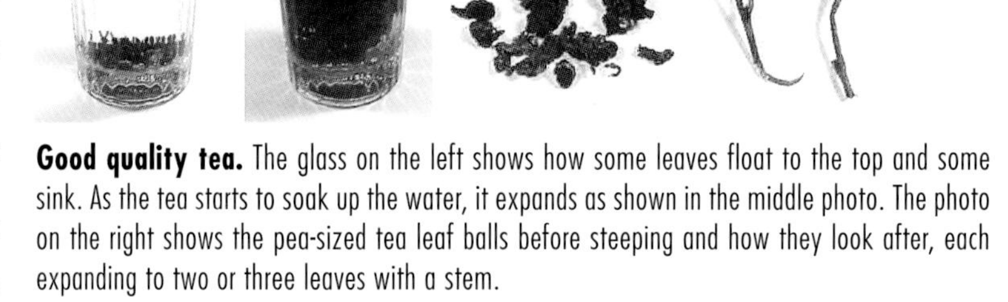

Good quality tea. The glass on the left shows how some leaves float to the top and some sink. As the tea starts to soak up the water, it expands as shown in the middle photo. The photo on the right shows the pea-sized tea leaf balls before steeping and how they look after, each expanding to two or three leaves with a stem.

Tea contains very complex chemicals, so never take medications with tea; it may cause an adverse reaction.

Reality Check

It was a nice visit and I received many packages of tea as departing gifts. One of the packages contained a famous award-winning tea, which I gave to my 99-year-old uncle. He was very happy to get it, and he held it in his hand for a long time. But for most people, the Taiwanese way of serving tea is not practical. Years ago, I learned another method from Chinese soldiers, and it is still a most popular way to drink tea. It is simple and practical.

Install an instant hot water system underneath the kitchen sink. The water should be charcoal filtered; or alternatively, you can heat a tall, clear glass of water in the microwave (if you use a colored or opaque glass or a coffee mug, the glass or mug tends to heat up more than the water). Add one to two tablespoonfuls of tea leaves to the tall glass with hot water. As you see in the above photos, some leaves float to the top and some sink. As the tea starts to soak up the water, it expands. The photo on the right shows tea leaves before and after expansion.

Start to sip it slowly in just a minute. It will be hot, but hopefully not too hot. The tea leaves may bother you at first, but the initial aroma is fantastic. I don't use a cover or fancy thermal cup because they tend to over-steep and make the tea taste too strong. Instead, I repeatedly fill the cup with hot water and drink it all day using the same leaves. Every time hot water is added, it changes the taste, but it tastes good all day. Yes, the same tea leaves all day! The taste of the tea gets weaker as the day goes on, and caffeine intake over the day is limited. On hot summer days, I strain it to get a clear glass of tea without leaves and make iced tea. In this way, I drink enough water to keep my doctor happy. It is also practical and inexpensive; a pound of tea will last a long time.

On occasion, tea often needs to be more elegantly served, and in some situations, I prepare it that way too. It is easily done with a tea set, and most families have an adequate tea set. If you use fresh tea leaves instead of tea bags, and no sugar or milk, you will enjoy the incredible aroma and flavor of your tea.

Here is another way of making tea suggested by a tea maker: fill the teapot half full of tea leaves, then fill with boiling water. As the tea is consumed, just add more water to the pot. For the first three pots, start to pour the tea after steeping it for fifty seconds; for the fourth through the sixth pots, pour the tea in one-and-a-half minutes; and for the seventh and eighth pots, pour the tea in two minutes. You will notice that the flavor and aroma change with each pot.

Instead of drinking coffee all day long, it is easy to use your coffee cup to make real tea. All you need is tea and hot water. Recent studies have indicated that strong tea is also effective in weight control. To make strong tea, place the teapot or coffee mug on the coffee warmer hot plate, cover, and let it stand for a while. This will make strong tea; most substances within the tea leaves are brewed into the liquid. But beware; strong tea tends to stain your teeth.

Buy your tea in stores or on the Internet from suppliers who specialize in supplying tea to Asian markets. Good tea can be expensive, but it's worth the money, and if you make it as described above, it can be economical. A pound of tea can cost from a few dollars to hundreds of dollars. As the economy in Asia is booming, more people are willing to pay for good tea, so the finer quality teas are getting more expensive. Try a few varieties to find the one you like.

In the early days, green tea was dried, powdered, and then simply placed in hot

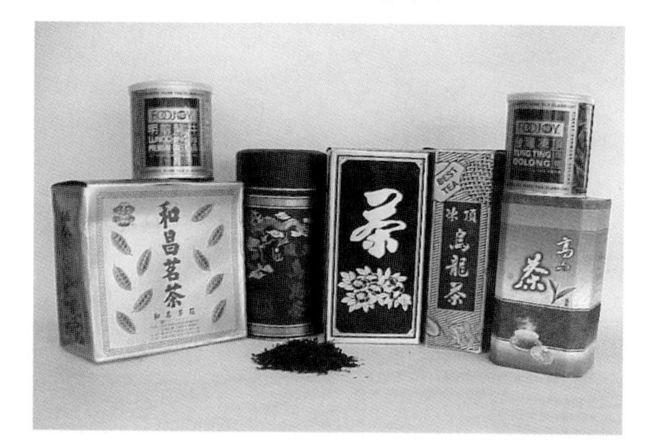

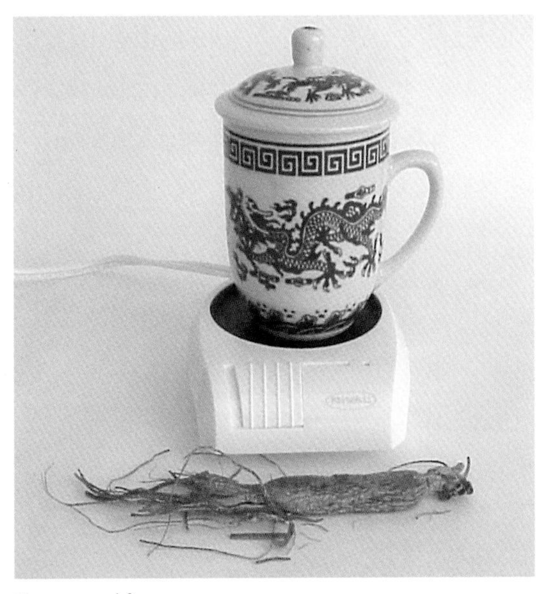

Ginseng used for tea

water to make tea. The Japanese learned how to do this from China around the seventh century, and they still drink it this way. In Japanese markets, you will find all sorts of teas that are prepared quite differently from the usual Chinese way.

A Word About Ginseng

Although ginseng is not tea, of course, it is a popular medicine throughout the world. There are about thirty varieties of the ginseng plant, and generally, ginseng is believed to nourish 'chi,' that is, invigorate your mind and body. Each variety has its specific medicinal value; for example, Korean ginseng is hot and strong, and Wisconsin ginseng is mild and excellent for general-purpose use. Wisconsin ginseng is known as American ginseng and is the most popular ginseng for everyday medicinal use. It is available in most Chinese markets.

Most people use ginseng like tea leaves. Instead, buy sliced ginseng and place three to six pieces in a coffee cup filled with boiling water. Let it sit covered for a few minutes. Just like the tea, keep adding hot water. The tea becomes weaker throughout the day as you add water, and eventually, you'll decide when you are finished with it. Ginseng tea is medicinal tea, nice to drink during cold and damp days. Personally, I drink it only occasionally, while I enjoy real tea everyday.

Folk Wisdom

Asian tradition holds that the host should not point the teapot spout at a guest, since that is a bad omen for friendship. Folklore tells us that tea dissolves fat; it is 'sharp,' so if you are undernourished or underweight (we all wish), you should not drink tea. Tea has been used in fingerbowls to cleanse fingertips after eating. Dishes cooked with tea as part of the ingredients will not spoil as quickly. Tea increases your mental alertness and relaxation at the same time. An offer of a cup of tea is, therefore, like an invitation to relax and enjoy the here and now for what it is.

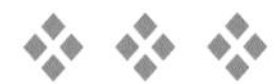

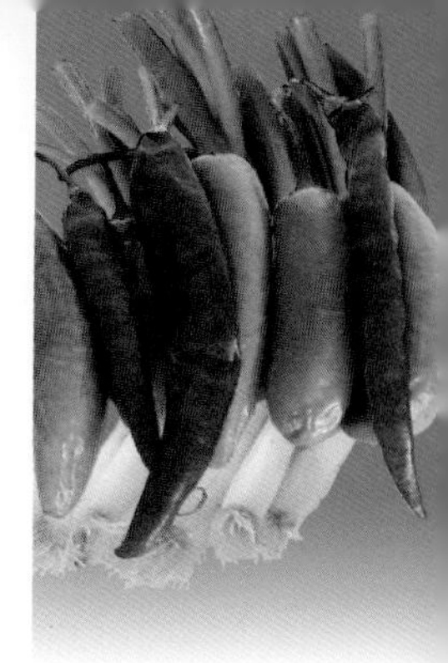

Chapter 9

Herbs and Spices

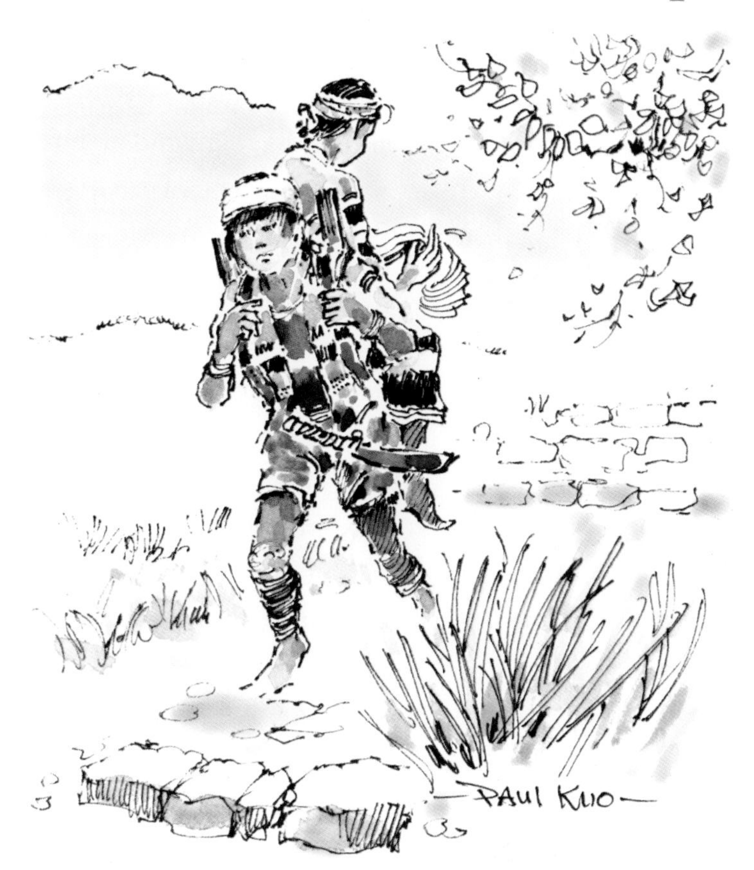

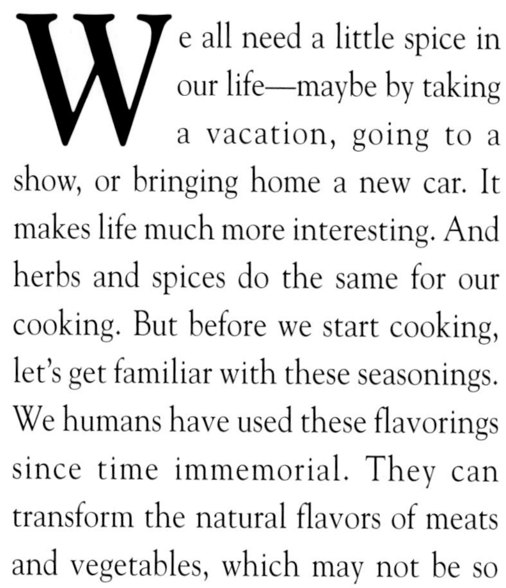

We all need a little spice in our life—maybe by taking a vacation, going to a show, or bringing home a new car. It makes life much more interesting. And herbs and spices do the same for our cooking. But before we start cooking, let's get familiar with these seasonings. We humans have used these flavorings since time immemorial. They can transform the natural flavors of meats and vegetables, which may not be so tasty alone, and also add to nutrition, as for example, the high vitamin C content and medicinal properties of paprika. In addition to making food taste good, they can help bring it into a proper yin/yang balance as well. They help us digest and absorb foods better—as, for example, ginger root, which is proven to help digestion.

Herbs and spices are typically concentrated, and they each contain a special complex of nutrients, and also some of the trace elements we need for ideal health. In fact, they may contain food elements that scientists have not yet identified, but which contribute to our health. Many American cooks use few spices—just seasoned salt, pepper, garlic salt, and maybe Italian seasoning. We are mostly familiar with the seasonings in processed foods, but by the time that food gets to us, the spices have lost their potency during processing and storage. It's not hard to expand our repertoire, however, and learn to use a wider variety of flavors in our food.

In this chapter, we look at American herbs and spices, and Asian flavorings, too. You will find most of these American herbs throughout European cuisine as well. Asian spices unique to Chinese cooking are not easily available unless you live near an Oriental market or can find them on the Internet.

Instead of using dried and processed herbs or spices, use them fresh whenever possible. To prepare fresh herbs for use, wash them and then holding the leaves or sprigs together in a bunch, chop coarsely and continue chopping to desired fineness. Fresh herbs lose their aroma and flavor quickly. To keep fresh for several days, trim the ends off the stems and place in a tall glass of cold water with a pinch of sugar, and then place them in the refrigerator. To revive wilted sprigs, moisten them with a fine mist of water and chill briefly.

You can buy fresh herbs at the grocery store, but they're so easy to grow. Even if you only have a window box, you might want to plant a bit of parsley, dill, basil, and other herbs for their beauty, aroma, and great taste in your cooking.

American Spices

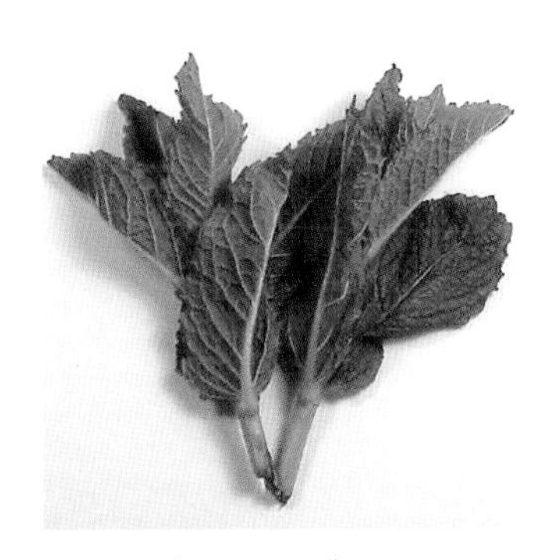

Basil. People often think of basil as an Italian herb, for instance the key ingredient in pesto sauce, but I think it goes with just about anything. You can sprinkle it generously, along with garlic powder and oregano, on skinned chicken parts and simmer them gently in a water-sherry mixture for an incredible, low-fat, tasty meat dish. I add it to most soups, stews, and sautés. Basil is the essential complement to tomato dishes; in fact, many people grow tomatoes and basil beside each other.

Bay Leaves. There are two main varieties of bay leaves: Turkish and Californian. The Turkish variety has a more subtle flavor.

Fresh bay leaves are superior to dried leaves, which have just a fraction of the flavor of the fresh leaves. They're very hard in texture, so you need to take them out before you serve a dish. They give that rich, meaty, brothy taste to simmered foods including soups and stews. They also add a rich bouquet to bean dishes; I especially like bay leaves simmered with white beans. When you slow-simmer meats, bay leaves add dimension and flavor.

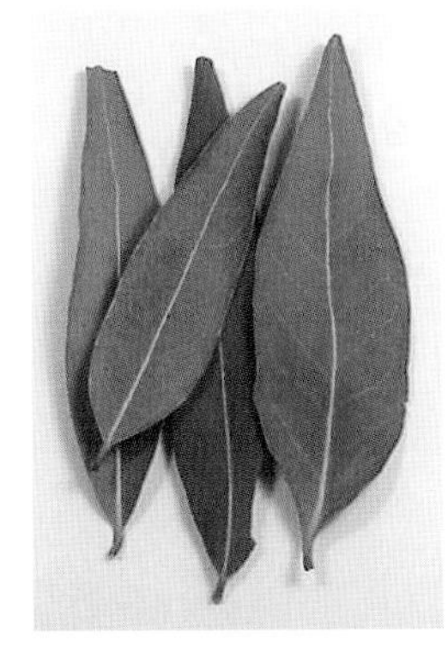

Cayenne Pepper (also known as Red Pepper). Health-food enthusiasts use cayenne pepper in just about every dish, but there's wisdom there; it's said to be good for the heart. You need to use it *very* gently, yet a few grains added to stewed meats, soups, and simmered dishes give a dimensionality and fullness you might like. Use it with a slightly (*very* slightly) more generous hand in egg dishes and bean dishes.

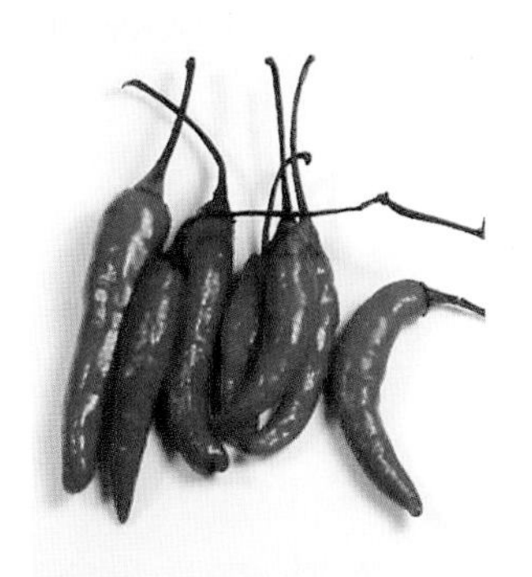

Chili Powder. This is actually a blend of several spices including chili, cumin, garlic, and sometimes other ingredients, with or without salt. Recent studies show that eating chili powder helps with menopausal symptoms. Use it in beans, Mexican or Southwestern dishes, and in smaller amounts as a flavor enhancer in soups and stews.

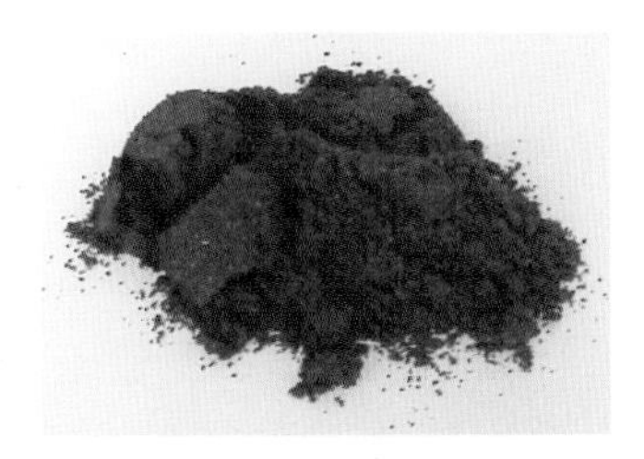

Chilies, Whole. There's a whole world of chili peppers out there—you can get a feel for this if you visit a Mexican store or the Mexican section in the grocery store. If you are cooking pinto beans or other beans, consider adding a few whole chilies to the pot. Fish them out when you're finished, and you'll have a nice chili flavor without that hot pepper bite. The big, flat chilies add a particularly nice flavor while the smaller chilies are slightly hotter. The smaller, whole chilies are sometimes used in Chinese stir-frying.

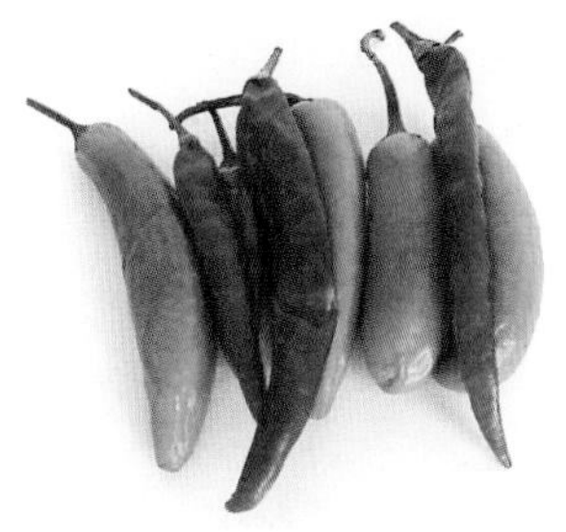

Chives. Related to the onion and leek, the delicate, hollow stalks resemble grass and taste like mild onion. Chives are an ingredient in *fines herbs*, which the French add to savory dishes. Cooking will diminish their flavor, so add to your dish at the last moment. If using as a garnish, add just before serving because cut chives can turn bitter. Chives are a good complement to potatoes, carrots, and green beans.

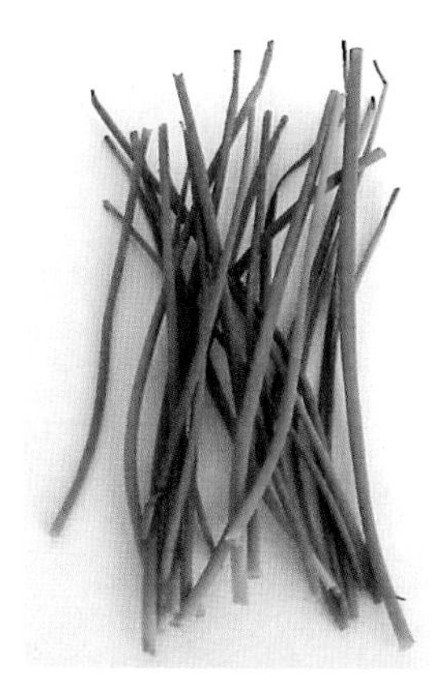

Cinnamon. Most people think of apple pie when they smell cinnamon. The sweet, nutty flavor of cinnamon is distinctive. It is the ultimate comfort aroma. Cinnamon sticks are often used in warmed winter drinks or as a flavoring for iced tea. You can slice peeled apples and gently stew them with a bit of sugar and cinnamon for a great side dish or dessert. In addition to its familiar uses in baking, cinnamon is simmered with lamb or chicken in the Middle East and is also used in Southeast Asia with meat dishes.

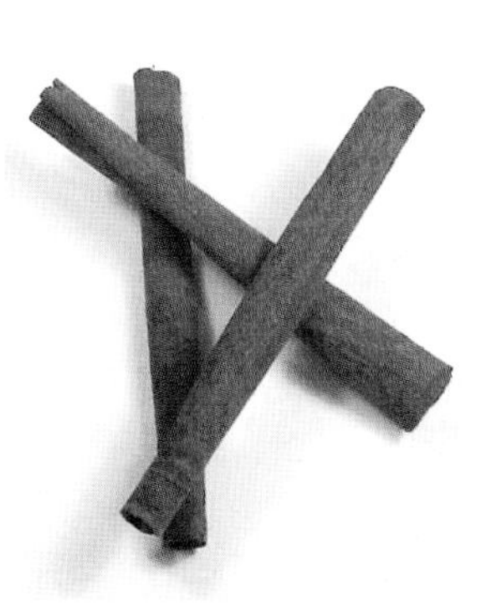

Curry Powder. Like chili powder, this is a blend of many spices. It is sometimes quite hot and sometimes a little sweet; there are actually many varieties. It's mostly used in rice dishes and in sauces to be served *over* rice. Experiment until you find a flavor your family likes.

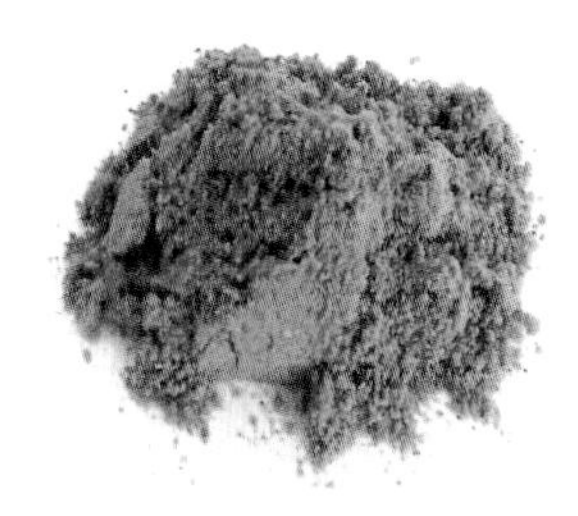

Dill. Dill's feathery, fern-like leaves are aromatic and tasty in sauces, dips, and soups. Use the seeds in salad dressings, casseroles, or soups, and use dill leaves in dips, vegetables, and for fish. Dill is soothing to the nerves—a good food-medicine.

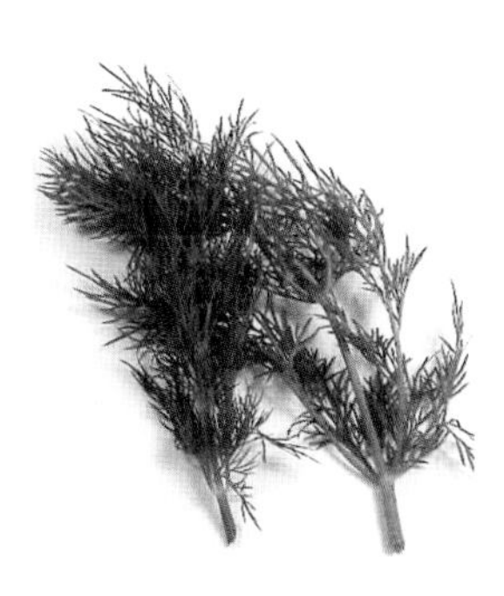

Horseradish. Aggressively spicy when its freshly peeled and grated, horseradish root releases an aroma so pungent that it brings on tears. Its strength fades quickly after grating, so use it immediately. This is mostly used as a garnish for stewed or grilled meats. You can mix it

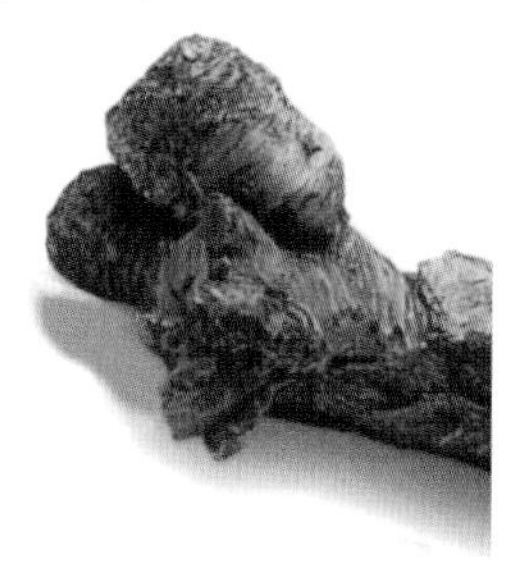

with mayonnaise to cut the hot taste. Horseradish is used to clear the sinuses, which you will immediately experience if you take more than just a pinch.

Marjoram. Marjoram is a member of the mint family and closely resembles oregano in flavor. Sometimes people use it interchangeably with oregano, although they are totally different plants. It tastes like a gentle, mild oregano. You can add it to soup, stews, veggie dishes, and most meat.

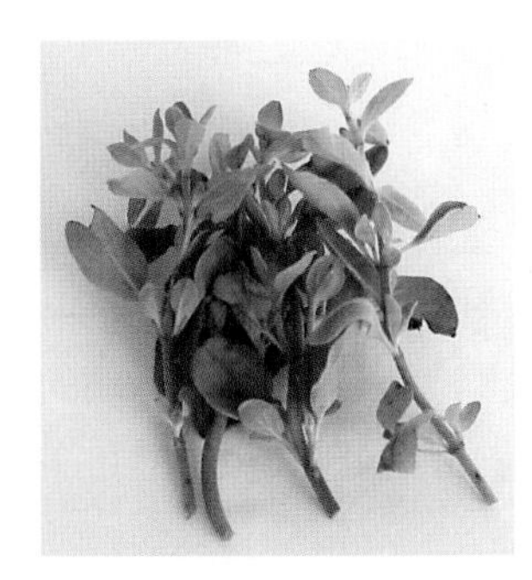

Mint. Although there are twenty-five varieties of mint, the two most commonly used mints are Peppermint and Spearmint. Peppermint, the more pungent of the two, has bright-green leaves with purplish stems. Spearmint has either dark green leaves or green-gray leaves.

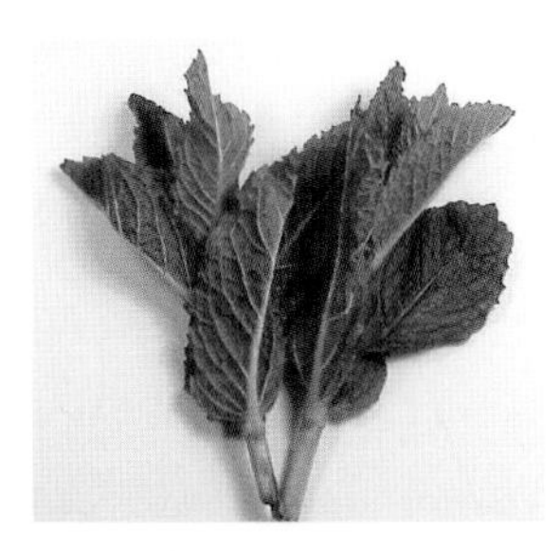

Mint is great with vegetables such as peas, potatoes, and carrots, or add half a handful of coarsely chopped mint leaves to salad greens. A good lamb marinade combines mint, raspberry, vinegar, soy sauce and garlic. Use mint in teas, soups and desserts. A great garnish, mint complements the flavors of a fruit salad. Mint is used by some people to soothe an upset stomach.

Nutmeg. Most people think of eggnog when they smell nutmeg. It's a common baking spice usually combined with cinnamon. Nutmeg is actually the seed of a tree, and you need to grate it before use. It's sold as a powder, but for a real culinary experience, buy some whole nutmeg and grate it on the fine side of a grater. You can try a little of this spice sprinkled over fish or chicken for a different taste.

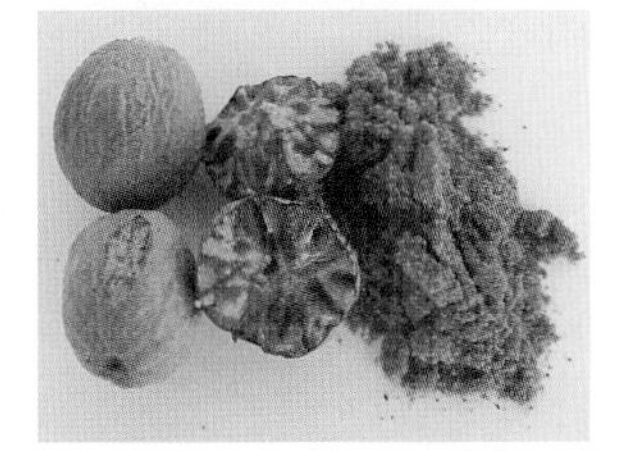

Oregano. Strong and spicy, oregano is an all-purpose herb. There are two varieties of oregano: Mediterranean and Mexican. Mediterranean oregano is milder, while Mexican oregano is used in hot, spicy dishes. Oregano is good in most meat and vegetable dishes. It adds to the fullness and richness of just

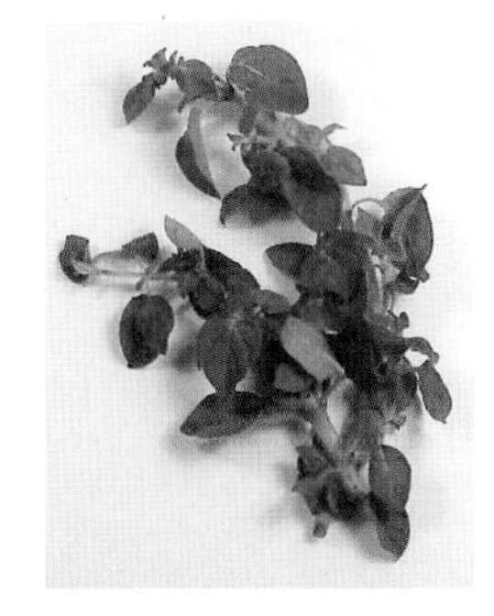

about any savory dish. It's mostly associated with Italian and Mexican cooking, but I use it for all styles.

Paprika. This is a member of the cayenne pepper family, but is *much* milder. It has one of the highest vitamin C contents in the whole plant kingdom, so it's a nice addition to almost any dish. Sprinkle it on top of casseroles, vegetables, and meat dishes for a gentle sparkle of flavor.

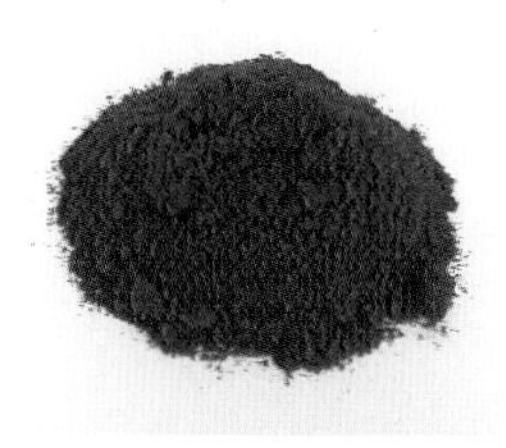

Parsley. There are two varieties of parsley: curly and flat-leaf. Parsley is much more than a garnish. Parsley is one of four, *fines herbs* that French chefs use to flavor their savory soups and sauces. It's so easy to grow parsley and have it fresh for cooking. If people would eat the pretty parsley garnish at the side of their plate, it would help their health. It's high in vitamin C and A, yet its mild taste goes with almost anything. I like to chop it and add it at the last few minutes to soup, vegetables, meat dishes, and as a garnish to salad dishes.

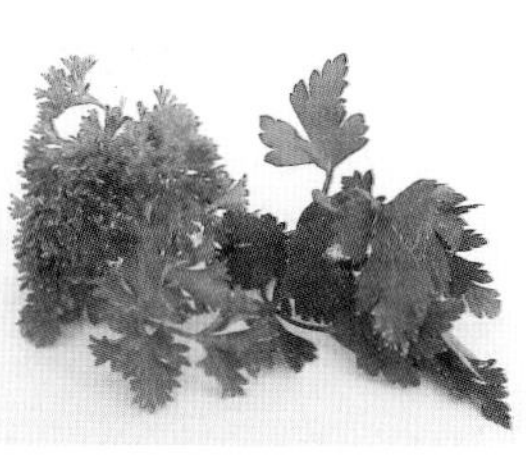

Peppercorns (and Ground Pepper). You can find pepper on just about every table in the nation. Most people buy ground pepper, but you will change that once you taste fresh, ground pepper. Pepper grinders are inexpensive and can last a long time. Black peppercorns are the immature seeds from the tree, while white peppercorns are the mature seeds.

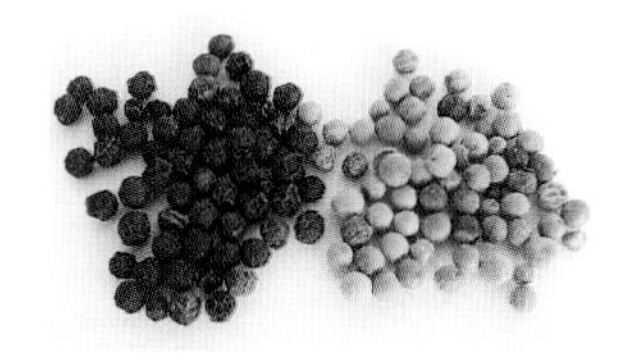

Poppy Seeds. Some say that eating poppy seeds can give you a positive drug test for opium since they are from the same family. Use them in baking (as in poppy seed muffins) or try adding them to the filling of tarts. They're a nice garnish for many dishes and are surprisingly delicious mixed in buttered noodles.

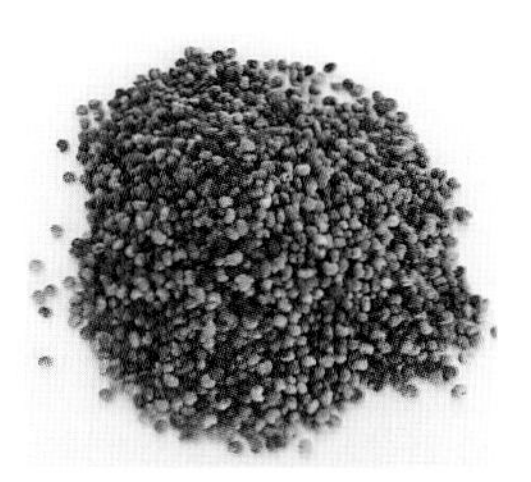

Rosemary. This has a very distinct flavor, so it can take a while to get used to it. It's amazing on roasted lamb (with garlic). It's also wonderful tossed with olive oil and garlic when roasting red, new potatoes. Rosemary is a

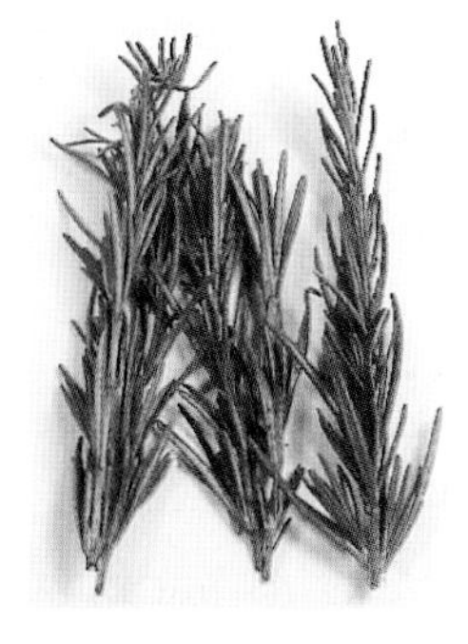

lovely herb to grow in your garden in temperate climates.

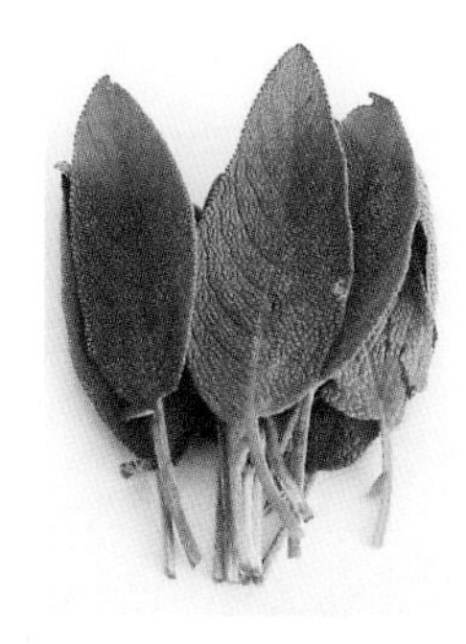

Sage. Sage has the pungent flavor of musty mint. Although most people may have sage in their pantries, they only use it around holidays for poultry dressings. It has a very distinctive flavor, so it's not for generous, everyday use. In addition to dressings, it's good with pork, poultry, and fish. It's another one of those medicinal herbs, an antiseptic.

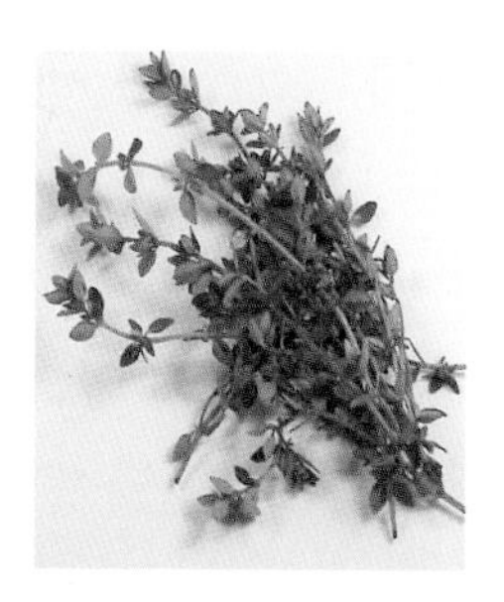

Thyme. This herb has a deeper, less sweet flavor than the commonly used basil and oregano, and it's another multi-use herb as well. Thyme, with its fragrant minty, lightly lemon aroma, is used in everything from chewing gum to cough syrup. Add it to your soups, stews, and meats. It blends well with most herbs, and it's especially nice with garlic.

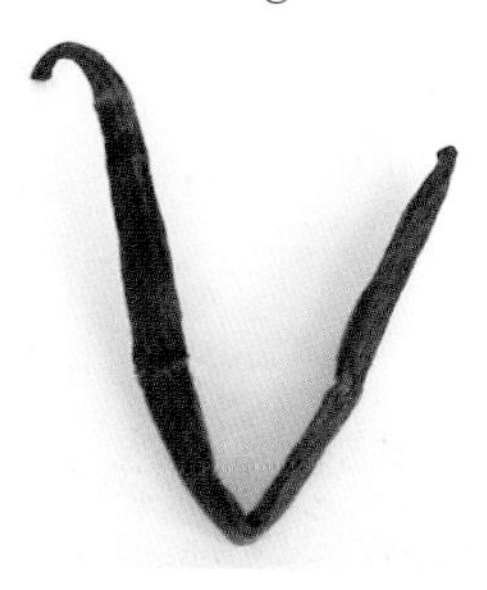

Vanilla. Just about everyone knows the flavor of vanilla. Try to buy the real vanilla rather than the imitation, it has a nicer flavor and it's healthier. In addition to its wide use in desserts, you can add a smidgen to sauces for meat to smooth out the flavor.

Asian Spices and Sauté Seasonings

Soy Sauce. Although you can buy only a few types at the usual American grocery store, there are actually many different varieties of soy sauce, most of which are very salty. Soy sauce mixes—such as teriyaki sauce, for example—are less salty and have unique flavors. Personally, I like to use teriyaki sauce since it has a good flavor for cooking, as well as tasting good when poured over foods at the table.

Every Asian ethnic group has its own favorite soy sauce. The Taiwanese like a special soy sauce, which is thick, less salty,

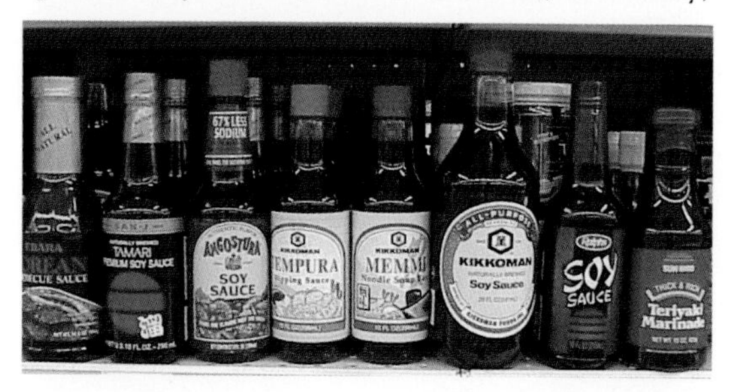

and slightly sweet. Most Americans like to use soy sauce on rice, but I prefer to serve the rice plain or use teriyaki soy sauce for better flavor.

If you use soy sauce on vegetables, it will discolor them. It's good in meat and fish dishes, or in mixed dishes containing meat and vegetables.

Ginger Root. Although it is not common in American cooking—except in desserts—ginger root is the most widely used spice in Asian dishes. It has a unique strong flavor and a slightly tingling hot taste, very different from the taste of hot chili peppers.

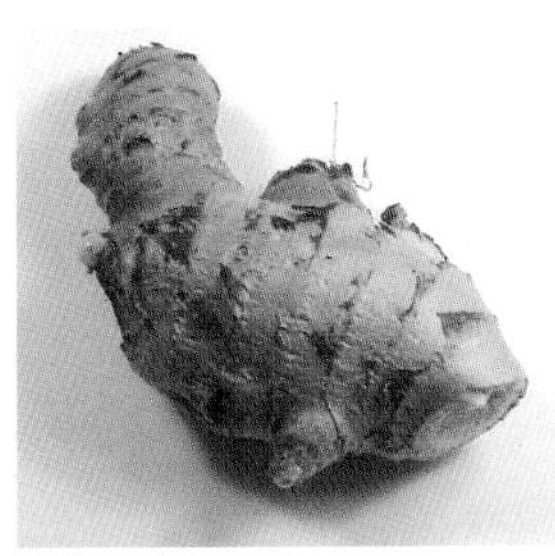

Ginger is rich in vitamins A and C, and it can soothe an upset stomach and kill harmful microorganisms that may contaminate food. It reduces blood cholesterol and prevents blood clots from forming. It also has anti-tumor and anti-cancer properties. Warm ginger broth sweetened with a little honey will soothe the symptoms associated with colds, especially a sore throat.

To make ginger tea, boil a dozen thin slices of gingerroot in three to four cups of water over low heat for about ten to twenty minutes, strain and sweeten with honey, and then drink it warm. It has warm outward energy, which helps to expel phlegm. In addition, clinical studies have proven ginger to be an effective anti-nausea remedy for motion sickness or pregnancy-related morning sickness. Small amounts of ginger root in our cooking may help protect us from many diseases.

In cooking, ginger root can be used to season almost any dish: meat, seafood, and vegetables. It can ameliorate strong flavors in particular foods. Older ginger is stronger, and used for cooking or as medicine. Young ginger is milder and is often served pickled with vinegar and sugar. This young, pickled gingerroot is served very thinly sliced in sushi bars in Japanese restaurants; the first dish served before the sushi. You can eat it to cleanse the palate between courses to get the true flavor of a new dish. This is especially true when eating raw fish or different varieties of seafood.

Ginger can also be thin-sliced or shredded for cooking. The skin is very thin; and it can be brushed or scraped off before cooking. Professional chefs can cut ginger into fine threads. It's not important to struggle to make tiny slices though; it doesn't affect the end result much. If you are going to stew ginger with meat, just mash it without cutting it into pieces. Grated gingerroot is generally mixed with soy sauce, teriyaki sauce, vinegar, or other sauces to pour over vegetables and as a dip for dumplings, meats, or in salad dressings.

Garlic. Garlic is a familiar ingredient in many styles of cooking, especially Italian

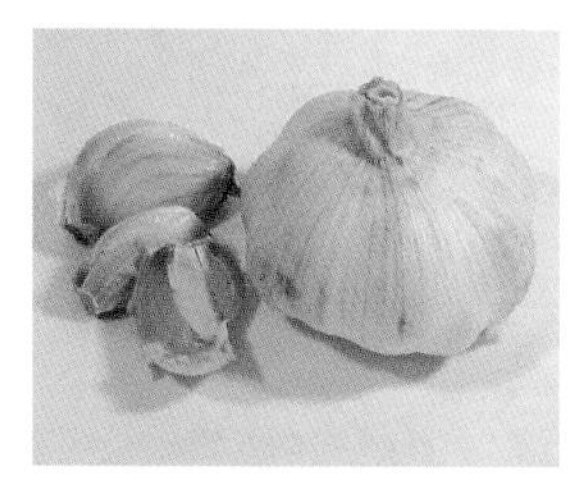

dishes. The health benefits of garlic are very well established in scientific research. It reduces bad cholesterol, increases good cholesterol, lowers blood pressure, and helps reduce blood clotting. It is an important flavoring in Chinese cooking, too.

Most cooks trim the stem end to release the paper shell over the garlic, which can then be peeled off. You can also smash the garlic and peel off the covering. If you cook it whole in a dish, mash it lightly to release the flavor. Most cooks mince it or put it through a special garlic press to get tiny pieces. You can also buy fresh, chopped garlic in a jar. This retains its flavor nicely and is ready whenever you are.

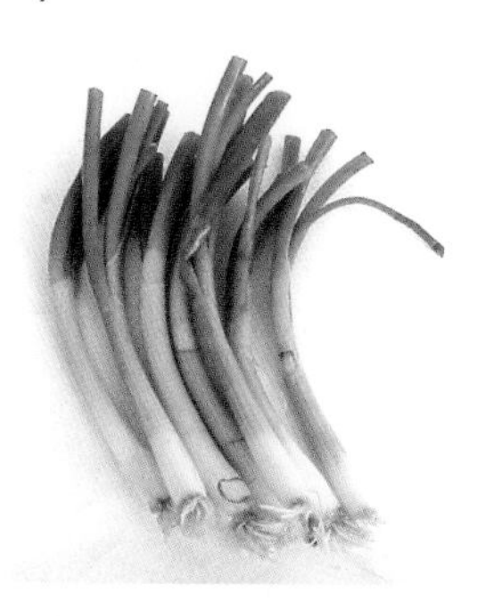

Green Onions. Green onions and shallots are fresh green members of the onion family with medicinal properties similar to garlic. Shallot is similar to green onion, except that it is a mature, dried bulb. In Asian cooking, most dishes contain onions, but they are very seldom eaten raw. For stir-frying, both green onions and dry onions can be cut into quarter inch strips or they can be chopped. Shallots have a slightly different flavor and are normally chopped to cook with meat dishes.

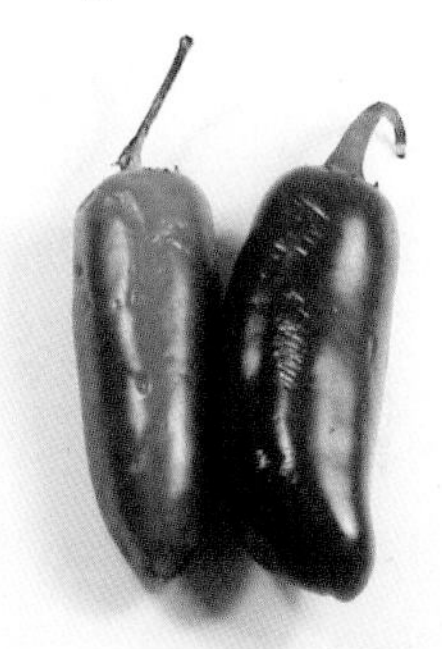

Jalapeño. Jalapeño also has excellent nutritional value. It has a nice green color that improves the appearance of light-colored dishes such as cabbage. Jalapeños have a delicious, hot taste, but if you don't like food very hot, remove the seeds and veins for less heat. Jalapeños are good in any stir-fry combination, especially stir-fry with meat.

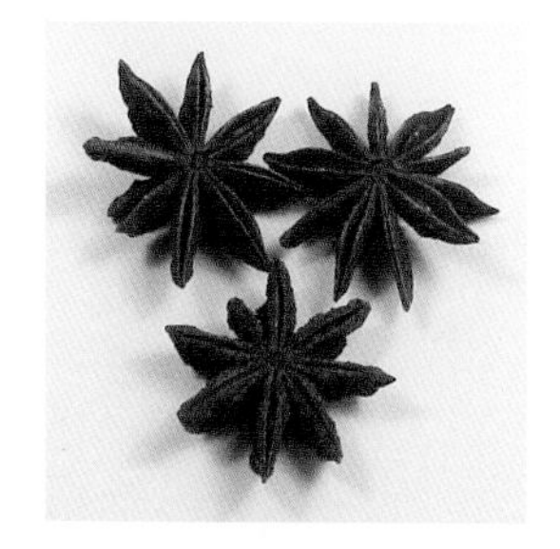

Star Anise. Star anise is a member of the parsley family. The seed has a unique, aromatic fragrance used for flavoring meat dishes in Chinese cooking. The unique smell in Chinatown town barbecue restaurants is partly the fragrance of anise seeds. It's also used as medicine for reducing intestinal gas. Star anise is very good for stewing, baking, or barbecue meat dishes including poultry. It adds a special fragrance and a unique, sweet taste.

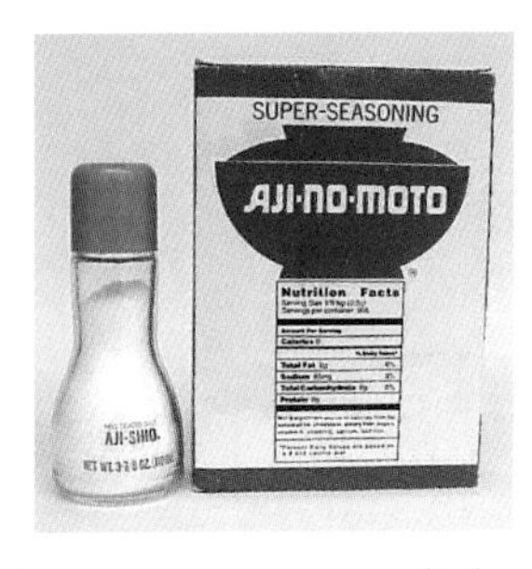

MSG. This is one of the most popular seasonings used in Asian cooking. Japanese and Taiwanese particularly like it. MSG is used in almost every dish, vegetables, meat, soup, and more. For more information about MSG, see Chapter 5, 'Glory Days of MSG.' If you're not used to MSG, you may not taste it at all, or you may not like it. If you use it, do so in moderation.

Fortunately, all of these herbs and spices are inexpensive and not hard to find in most grocery stores. See if you can find them, and keep them on hand for your everyday cooking. It helps to keep your dried spices in the freezer because they retain their flavor and strength much better and longer.

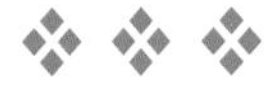

PART FOUR

Serve It Up

Do Americans eat any differently from their European cousins? Consider that the average American is sixteen pounds heavier than the average European. While 15 percent of European adults are considered obese, 24 percent of American adults fall into that category. Since the majority of Americans are of European origin and the living standard in Europe is comparable to the American living standard, the disparity probably lies in the difference in diets. Europeans eat more traditionally with variety in their foods, while Americans are consuming a steady diet of modern, processed foods.

In days gone by, it was believed that children growing up in a family with many children were generally healthier than children from a smaller size family. In a large family, more foods were needed and served on the dinner table with little room for catering to individual tastes and preferences, thus resulting in a greater variety in the diet. One may also conclude that children in a large family not only ate a greater variety of foods, they also learned to accept and like a varied diet. Demanding and getting only what they like to eat, on the other hand, can easily spoil children from a small family. Their food preferences and choices grow narrower and narrower.

Today, our family size is small and life hectic, so the convenience of processed food limits our food selections and nutritional sources resulting in an unbalanced diet. The counterbalance to this downward spiral is to expand our dietary habits to include a better variety of foods. Part Four of this book provides a winning strategy for a balanced diet in this modern world.

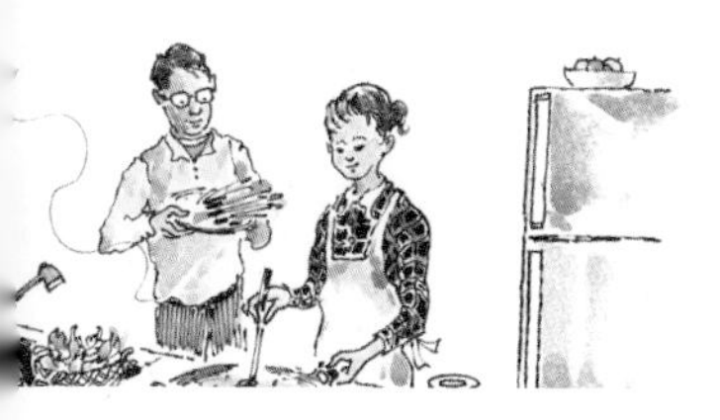

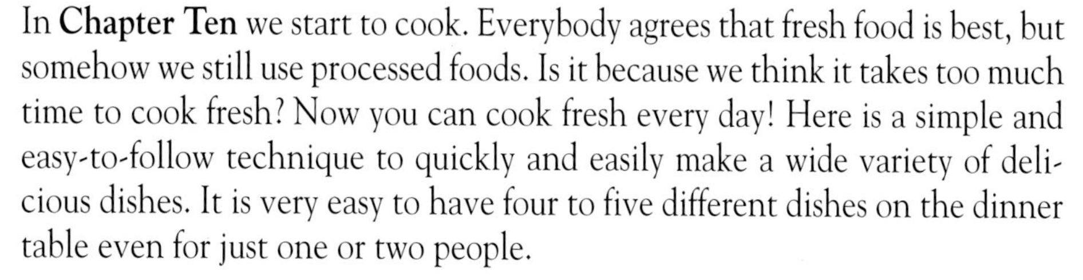

In **Chapter Ten** we start to cook. Everybody agrees that fresh food is best, but somehow we still use processed foods. Is it because we think it takes too much time to cook fresh? Now you can cook fresh every day! Here is a simple and easy-to-follow technique to quickly and easily make a wide variety of delicious dishes. It is very easy to have four to five different dishes on the dinner table even for just one or two people.

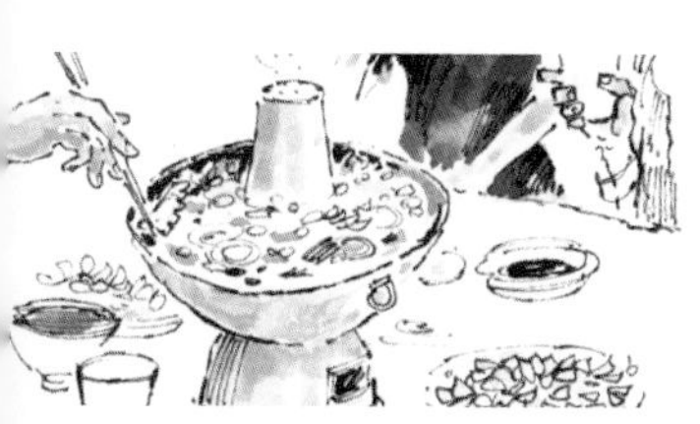

In **Chapter Eleven** we look at how our ancestors relied on foods that we hardly eat today, yet they're still very important for good health. Soup, porridge, and pickles were central to the daily diet in the past. Here we discuss *why* they're important and how to easily include them in our diets.

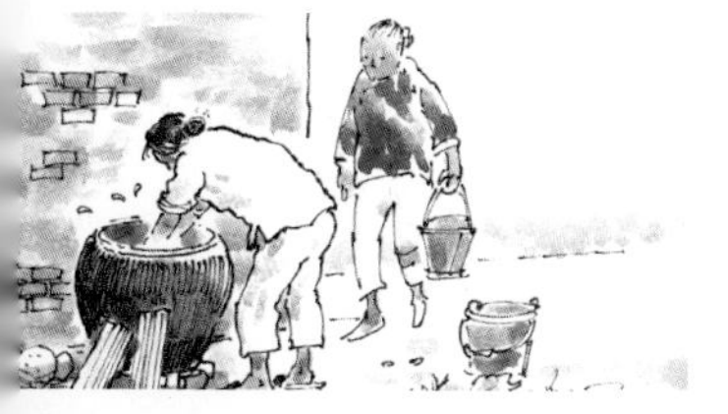

In **Chapter Twelve** we revisit the old traditional, fermented vegetables. Fermentation produces enzymes, which are antibiotic, anti-carcinogenic, help in digestion, and support the immune system. We will discuss what fermentation is and how to make fermented foods part of your dinner table.

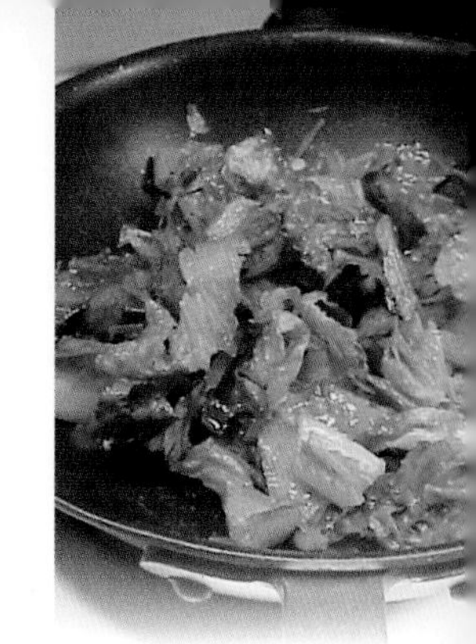

Chapter 10

Let's Start Cooking

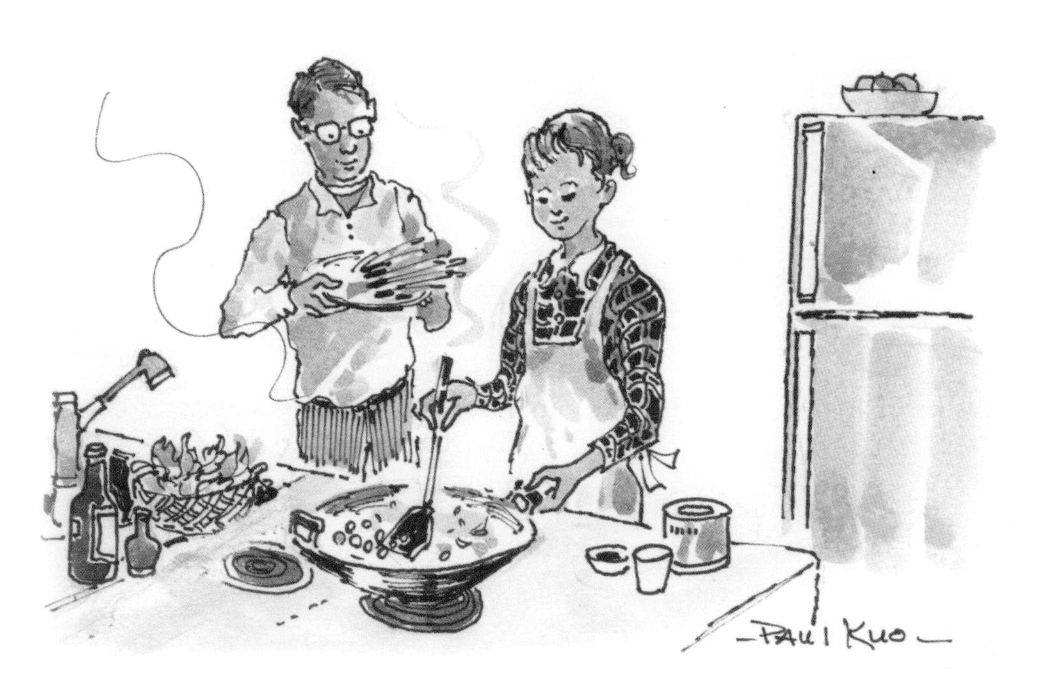

Most Americans are affluent enough to eat out regularly in restaurants, especially fast-food restaurants, even though we probably realize that restaurant food isn't the best for building good health. To be realistic, restaurants would never survive as a business if their menus were designed only for their customers' health. Most of us can't afford to hire a 'majordomo' to prepare a delicious, healthy meal for us. The only way to eat well everyday is to take care of ourselves.

Now that we have discussed the benefits of a simple fresh-food diet, you may be wondering how to put all this information to practical use from day to day, especially with a busy schedule. In this chapter, I'll tell you how. This is much more than some new diet; as you will see, it's really a way of life. With just a few simple changes in lifestyle, you'll enjoy a wide variety of foods that you cook fresh at home, easily, everyday.

Before you get started, I suggest that if you're married or living with someone, that both of you get a feel for the new information here, and that you get together on what changes are coming. Rest assured, though, that you will enjoy plenty of freedom because this way of cooking means total *individuality*. How your meal turns out—even starting out with the same foods—depends entirely on the cook. And today, the cook may be the man, the woman, or even the children in a family. It's fun to share the cooking and enjoy the variety. No matter who cooks, you're going to enjoy the diversity and improvement in your everyday food, as well as the benefit to your day-to-day health.

Eat a Variety of Food

If you eat a variety of food, you don't have to become overly concerned about what's healthy and what's not. You just eat less of the less-healthy foods, such as sweets and fats and highly processed foods, and you don't eat too much of anything. Contrary to popular opinion, it's important to eat some fat including animal fat; just don't overdo it. For example, we cook with olive oil and use good meat with the fat trimmed, which retains just enough animal fat for a balanced, healthy diet. For each meal, you'll prepare three or four dishes, but no special main dish, which is usually meat in the typical American diet.

In the following paragraphs, you'll find cooking techniques that allow you to cook good stuff everyday with the least amount of time and effort. I'm not giving you recipes here; what you're getting are techniques that allow you to cook a delicious meal quickly. You can vary the ingredients for different dishes; that way, you're eating something new everyday.

How to Cook Vegetables Essential for a Healthy Diet

Let's start with how to cook vegetables. Your mother probably told you, "Eat your vegetables," and even though kids don't always agree, most adults do. If you don't like veggies, it's likely you haven't tasted them properly cooked. In America, most people boil, steam, or bake vegetables (when they are not eating them raw), then season them with salt and pepper and butter. On the other side of the world, Chinese cooks have been stir-frying veggies for centuries. Stir-frying is quick, easy, and delicious; the veggies retain their fresh taste and their nutrients and are easy to digest. And believe it or not, it's not really 'frying;' it's more of a quick and delicious steaming technique.

Stir-frying can transform any vegetable into a meal. It's a good way to expand the variety of veggies in our diets. There's no specific rule to making a good stir-fry dish; however, there are some simple principles for stir-fry cooking.

Rice and Automatic Rice Cookers Again

First of all, you serve stir-fry with rice, so you need a rice cooker. I recommend that every family have a good automatic rice cooker. Buy one with steamer baskets and you can add some steamed dishes to the dinner table with minimum effort. Once you get accustomed to having fresh steamed rice with your dinner, you may never want to go back to eating store-bought bread.

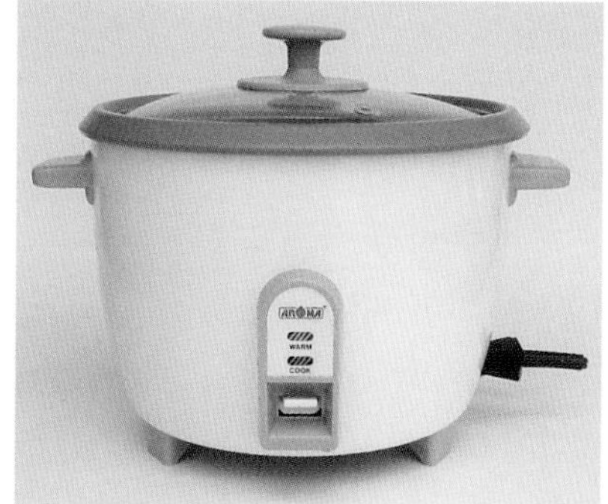
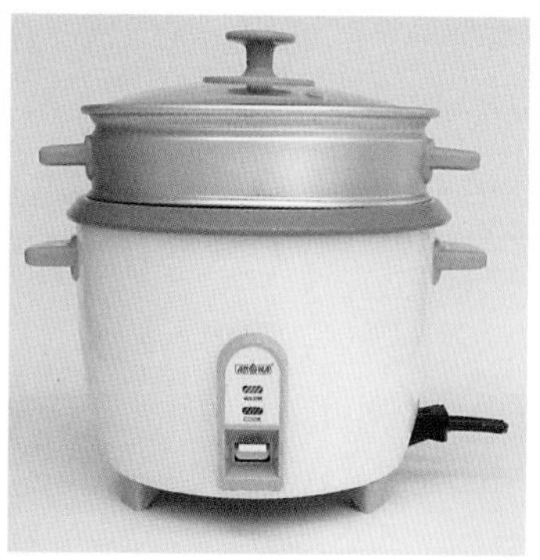

A rice cooker (left), and rice cooker with steamer (right).

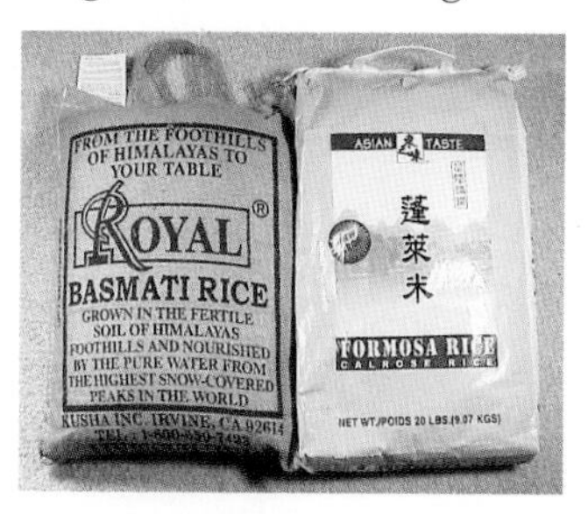

Although you can only purchase a few types of rice at most grocery stores, there are actually many delicious varieties of rice. *Formosa* rice is normally served in Japanese restaurants. It has a very soft texture and is somewhat sticky. *Jasmine* rice (*Basmati* rice) is the variety served in most Chinese restaurants. It has a nice aroma and is soft, but not sticky. It tastes like something between long grain rice and Formosa rice. This is good rice to use and it is available in most markets.

More About Cookware

What kind of pan do you need to stir-fry? As we mentioned before, a European stir-fry pan is ideal. The non-stick pan shown in the photo below (twelve-inch diameter, six-inch flat bottom, four inches high) works great. Your usual sauté pan is less ideal because of the low sides. Chinese woks really don't work well because of the round bottom. They're great for conventional Chinese stoves but not for our modern stoves.

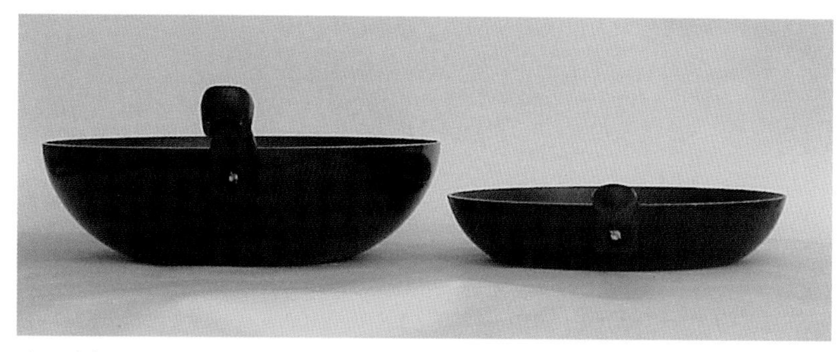

Above left is a European stir-fry pan and a sauté pan is shown on the right.

Basic Pantry Items

Make sure you have these items in your pantry: rice, flour, cornstarch, soy sauce, olive oil, wine, vinegar, pepper, salt, sugar, spices, star anise, MSG, and any of your favorite herbs. In addition, for initial seasonings, we need ginger, shallots, green onions, regular onions, jalapeño peppers, and garlic.

Most veggies are delicately flavored so they don't taste good with overly strong seasonings. You want to taste the natural flavor of the vegetables and not have them overpowered. However, in contrast to simple steamed vegetables, stir-frying gives veggies a unique flavor and a good yin/yang balance. Veggies are mostly yin, so you need to add yang somehow to balance the yin—which means adding something to give a warm and hearty taste to the vegetables. In stir-frying, this process is achieved by lightly frying some seasoning to warm the dishes. You know you have a balanced, wholesome dish when veggies taste fresh, delicious, and hearty at the same time. Your sixth sense will tell you when you have it right; after your meal, you'll feel satisfied and good.

The first step is to heat the pan, add a little olive oil (just enough to coat the bottom of the pan), add your seasonings, and stir them around for just a few minutes, just until they start to give out a delicious

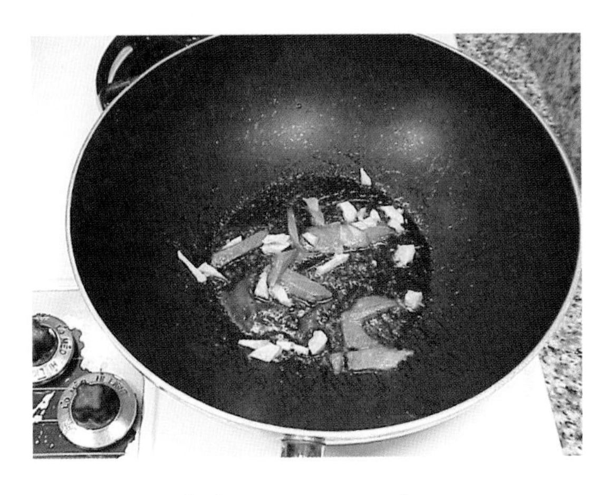

aroma. I call this 'sautéing' the seasonings.

This is one technique most Americans miss when they cook veggies, but it results in a well-balanced, delicious dish. This process adds yang to veggies; in other words, it gives them that warm savory taste. The heated oil slightly browns the seasonings—such as garlic or ginger—almost like deep-frying. Sautéing brings out a wonderful aroma and flavor. Use minced garlic, minced fresh ginger, onions, bacon/ham, and similar seasonings. If you use bacon, reduce the amount of oil. See the technique for stir-frying broccoli, below, for detailed instructions regarding spices, cooking times, preparation, etc.

In Taiwan, we enjoy another sauté ingredient: small shrimp and fish, which are dried and preserved for seasoning stir-fry and other dishes. When you cook veggies, the dried shrimp or fish provide a nice meaty, glutamate protein flavor to vegetables such as cabbage and cu-

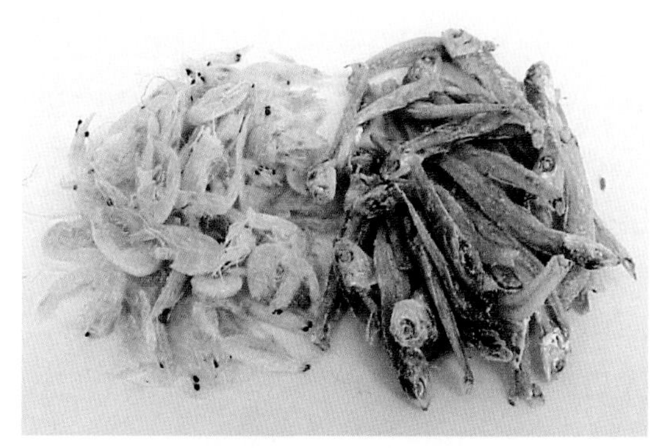

cumbers. This used to be the poor man's way to get protein.

As with most unfamiliar foods, some American friends love the taste and some won't even try it. We eat the whole shrimp and fish including the bone and shell, which provides natural minerals and nutrients that are not easy to get by eating other foods. No doubt, bacon is more popular, but for health, few will disagree that dried baby shrimp and fish is better for you.

Be careful when sautéing garlic because it browns quickly and can burn before you know it. If it turns dark and tastes odd or somewhat bitter, you'll know that you fried it too long or the heat was too high. When you begin your sauté this way, you get the benefit of the oil, which dissolves non-water-soluble nutrients and helps tenderize the veggies. Although the Chinese use this technique, you can also find it used all over the world. Stir-frying cooks ingredients quickly; so prepare them all beforehand.

An Example: Stir-Frying Broccoli

Instructions. Try this same method for stir-fried broccoli, but you can use the same technique for all veggies.

1. Use a sauté pan, 10 inches or more in diameter. Turn the heat high to preheat the pan, reduce to medium heat after the pan gets hot, and add 1 or 2 tablespoons of olive oil. Swirl it around in the pan.

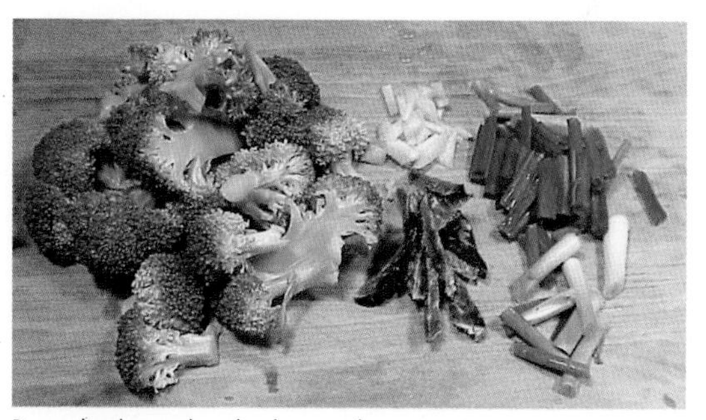
Broccoli, chopped garlic, ham and green onion

2. Add seasonings such as ham, bacon or garlic, which taste good with broccoli. Watch carefully so they don't burn and turn bitter. As soon as the seasonings are slightly browned, add the cleaned, cut broccoli, and stir a few times. Then reduce the heat, add 3 to 4 tablespoons of water, and cover.
3. Let the broccoli steam for less than a minute, add the green onion, and then check to make sure that there's a small amount of water in the bottom of the pan. Test the broccoli with a fork to see if it's tender enough. If

needed, add more water and let it steam longer until it tastes right to you. A clear glass cover works well to watch the veggies cook.

4. Salt and pepper to taste. When you taste this, you will love it; it's delicious and wholesome. If George Bush's chef knew how to cook vegetables like this, I am sure he would like broccoli!
5. Bacon is optional; cut 1 or 2 slices of bacon into 1/2-inch pieces and sauté with the garlic. Bacon increases the yang property of the dish. Since bacon is salty, be careful about how much salt you add. If you like the plain taste of broccoli and don't want the taste of the sautéed seasonings, don't add them. Another option is you can add some chicken or beef bouillon.

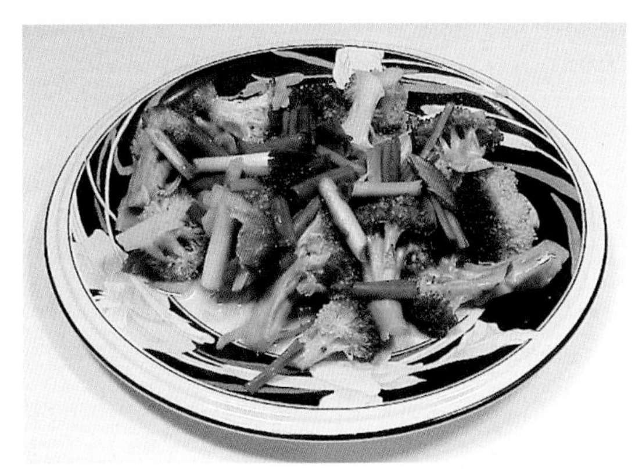

Simple healthy dish

Cooking is an art and you are the artist. Follow your own instincts; adjust the ingredients and portion sizes as you go along based on the number of individuals you are serving. Just remember that soy sauce can overwhelm the natural taste and color of the broccoli, so if you really want to add soy sauce, use teriyaki sauce instead; it is lighter and more flavorful.

The Sauce. The final step is the sauce. Add two tablespoons of cornstarch to one cup of water and mix well. At the last minute, add this mixture to the dish you are cooking. Stir in slowly, a bit at a time, until the cornstarch and water have changed the sauce to the desired thickness. It should not be too thick. Discard the rest of the starch-water mixture. The amount needed depends on how much liquid you are cooking with. Starch will bind up the liquid in the pan and reduce the volume of your sauce. Watch how the sauce thickens; too much of the cornstarch/water mixture will make the sauce too thick. If this happens, add more water, a little at a time, to thin it. Add a teaspoon of vinegar such as balsamic vinegar if you like, and it will give the sauce a special tangy flavor.

This quick stir-fry method gives a delicious flavor to broccoli with minimum cooking, which preserves nutrients. Broccoli cooked this way is easy to digest and is simply delicious. It is very different from our conventional way of eating broccoli, and it is a good basic dish for vegetarians.

With a little adjustment, this technique will cook most vegetables. Cauliflower, cucumbers, green beans, bell pepper, cabbage, eggplant, sliced carrots, celery, mustard greens, and most other vegetables can be stir-fried in this simple, delicious way. Use your imagination for various combinations. Just be sure that you check for tenderness every half-a-minute or less, and make sure the water doesn't boil away and burn your food. It is safer to use low to medium heat because high heat can easily burn the food. And clear, glass covers help you keep an eye on your veggies.

Just before serving, while the food is hot, you might place one or two slices of cheese on top of cauliflower, broccoli, or cabbage dishes, a nice touch for cheese lovers. For vegetables that need a longer cooking time to become tender such as carrots, turnips, daikon, heavy green-leaf vegetables, etc., it is not necessary to sauté the seasonings since a longer cooking time will dilute the sautéed spice flavor anyway, and most of the flavor transfers to the juice. For these heavier vegetables, simply boil together with bacon, ham, or any tasty meat, and let the veggies absorb the flavor from the meat.

Stir-frying is great for soft, tender leafy vegetables such as spinach, bok choy, and lettuce (yes, lettuce!). Just be aware that these vegetables have a high water content and will release water during cooking. Use a higher heat and cook the greens quickly, stirring constantly, to avoid sogginess. With spinach, for example, stir quickly until leaves are limp, then add salt and pepper, and remove from heat. If the leaves release much moisture, you know that you have cooked the leaves too long. After a little practice, you'll become an expert at this. You can mix different-colored leafy veggies, thin sliced carrots, and tomatoes for a delightfully colorful vegetable dish.

If prepared and cooked properly, this kind of cooking retains the original color and texture of your veggies. Everybody knows the soggy, gray look of overcooked vegetables. While you don't want to undercook, try not to overcook as well.

Although this method looks a lot like the conventional way to cook vegetables, I think you will be surprised at how absolutely delicious they are cooked this way. Your kids may finally start to enjoy their veggies!

General Guidelines

With a little practice, you will find your own individual way of cooking stir-fry and discover your favorite flavorings. However, I can give you a few general guidelines.

- Use garlic for most veggies and meats.
- Ginger and green onions are used for meat and seafood. Most people don't

combine ginger and garlic, but if you like the combination, try it.

- Don't use soy sauce to stir-fry veggies because it will darken your dish and change the flavor of the veggies. If you insist on soy sauce, use teriyaki soy sauce; it is lighter and more flavorful.
- You can add sliced green onions at the end of cooking for a pleasant green garnish.
- I particularly like plain veggie dishes cooked just right with a little MSG or a pinch of sugar added at the end to bring up the flavors.
- You can also add jalapeño at the end of cooking for a touch of spiciness. This adds warmth to the dish and makes the dish more yang.

Why Not Try Some New Veggies?

As the Asian population increases in America, many vegetables are appearing in the market that are not familiar to Americans. I'd like to introduce you to some of these new, delightful foods, which you may enjoy.

Daikon. Looks like an enormous white carrot. This Asian radish has a peppery, pungent but sweet, and fresh flavor. It contains *diastase*, an enzyme that aids digestion. It's easy to grow year round and can be found in most supermarkets. It is eaten

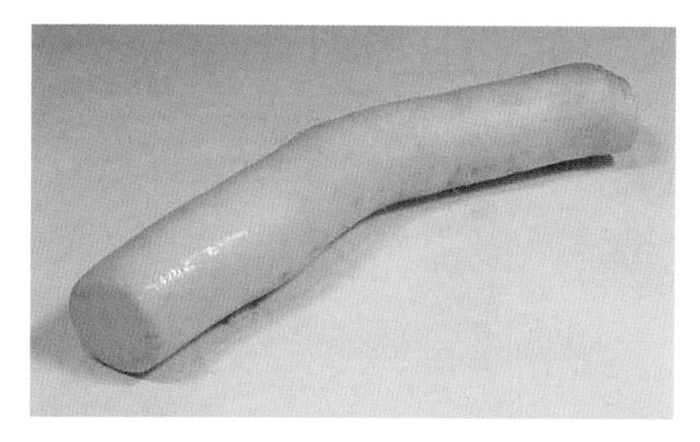

fresh, cooked with meat, pickled in kim chi and other pickles, and preserved by drying. It doesn't taste good uncooked. It tastes great cut into one-inch cubes and cooked with meat in soy sauce; this combination creates a very delicious flavor.

Chinese or Napa Cabbage. More tender and flavorful than common cabbage, this is one of the most popular vegetables among Asians. It's available year-round and is eaten stir-fried or in various pickles. It releases moisture when cooked,

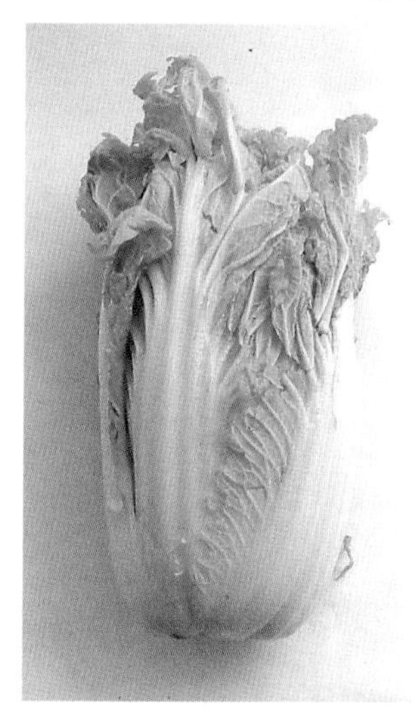

but tastes great and takes on a sweet flavor when simmered for a while. It is great to cook with a meat dish or in soup.

Chinese Broccoli and Chinese Mustard. Chinese broccoli, a green, leafy plant with small white flowers, is highly nutritious.

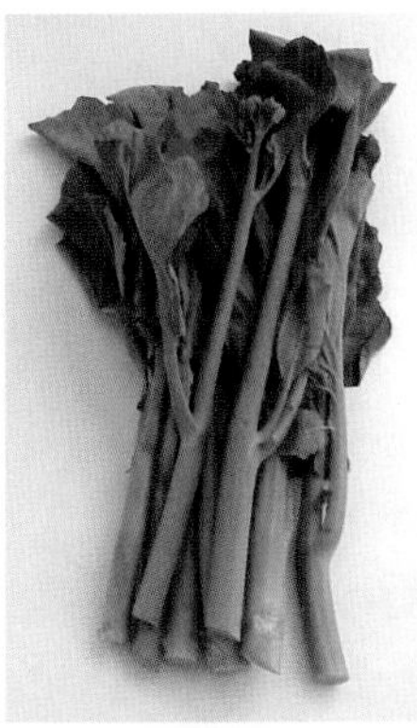

Chinese broccoli

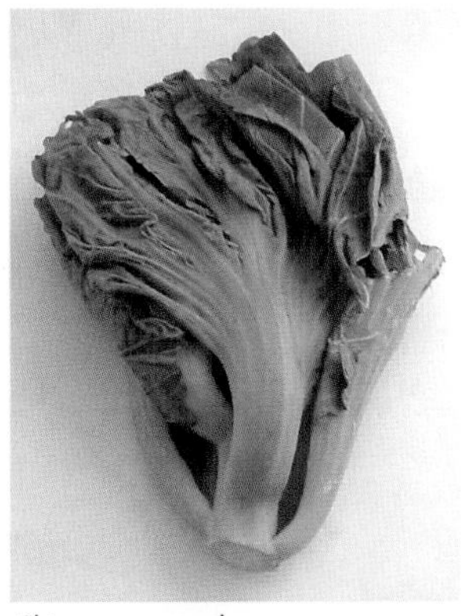

Chinese mustard

When cooked, the firm stem is tender, delicate, and full of flavor. High in nutrition, this is a vegetable you must try. It is the most popular dish in Chinatown. Chinese mustard has a stronger taste and flavor. It cooks like common cabbage. Both of these are very popular and believed to be highly nutritious veggies among the Chinese.

Bok Choy. Any veggie without a proper English name ends up being called 'bok choy.' They are all green and leafy, look and taste healthy, and stir-fry nicely.

Before cooking vegetables, be sure to wash them well using warm water, which removes more chemicals than cold water. Of course you want to remove the dirt and bugs (which can't hurt us, by the way), but also the chemicals (which can). Peel if needed and cut into one-inch pieces. For stir-frying root vegetables such as carrots, turnips, and yams, be sure to slice them thin.

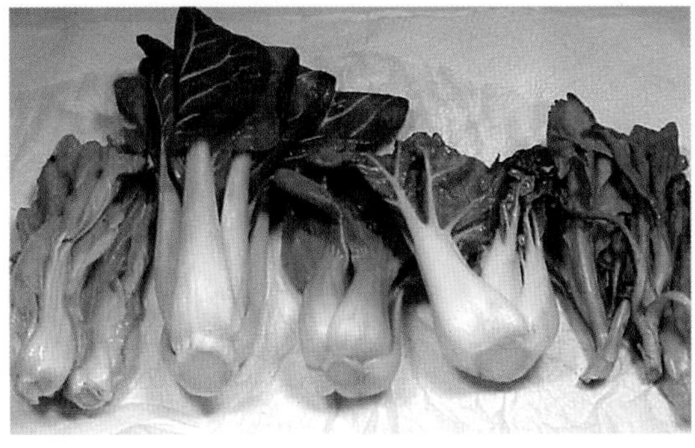

Samples of bok choy

Cutting Vegetables

Cutting veggies is simple common sense. You need to cut them to a size that is easy to cook and good for presentation, or simply looks appetizing. There are several ways vegetables are cut.

Coarse Cut. For stir-frying leafy vegetables, generally make this cut. Space the cuts about one-half inch to one inch.

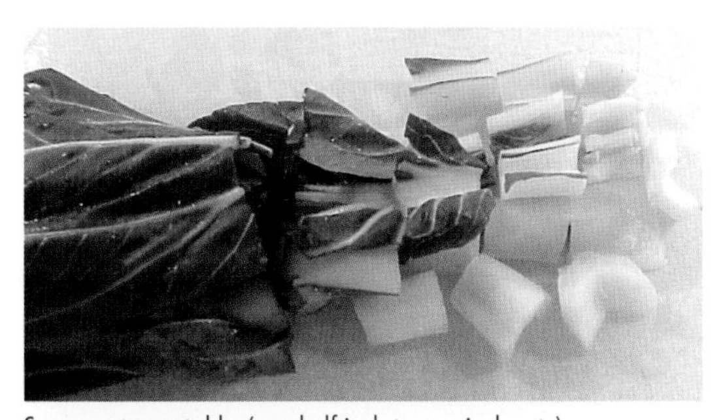

Coarse-cut cegetable (one-half-inch to one-inch cuts)

Medium Cut. This cut is for quick, stir-fry vegetables that are a little hardy and need short cooking times such as cabbages and bok choy. This cut is approximately one-quarter-inch in length.

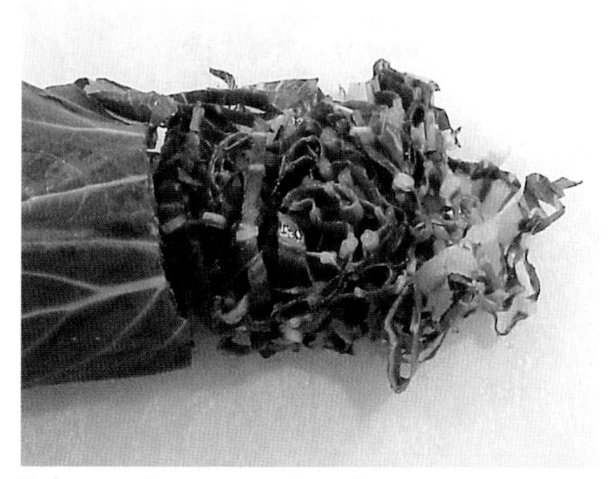

Medium cut: about a quarter of an inch.

Fine Cut. Cut fine for garnishing on top of dishes for a nice presentation.

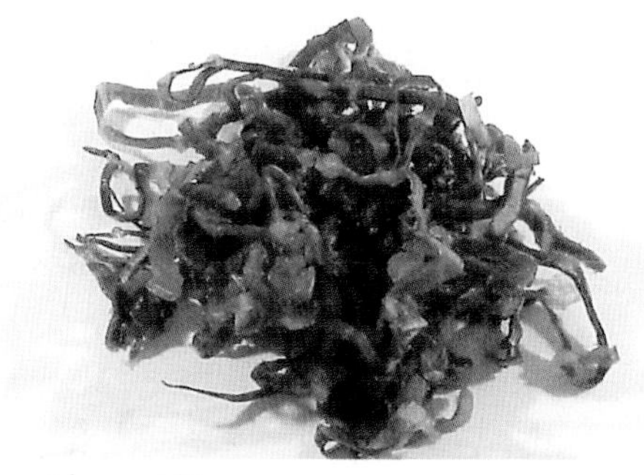

Fine cut for garnishing

Long Slice Cut. For carrots and green onions, this cut is for easy cooking and nice presentation. Carrots are cut in chunks, thin slices, and long strips.

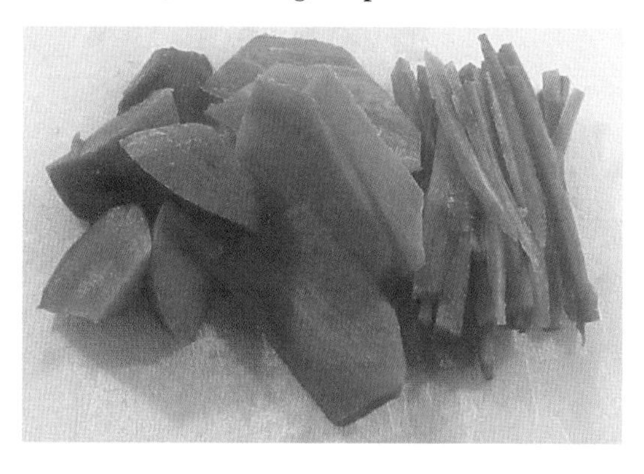

Prepared Fresh Veggies

As you probably know, preparing the veggies takes the most of your cooking time. You can often buy pre-cut vegetables for stir-frying at the supermarket, and there's nothing wrong with fresh, frozen veggies either. It is well documented that fresh, frozen vegetables retain most of the original nutrients. Just be aware that fresh, frozen vegetables are coated with a thin layer of water to protect them from frostbite, so they need a little less water during cooking. Frozen veggies come in many varieties and mixtures ready to stir-fry. You can either wash them first or simply place them frozen in a hot pan and let them cook. Fresh is always better, but keep on hand a good supply of frozen veggies for a healthy dish ready in minutes.

A Few Exceptions

With this simple technique, you can turn frozen veggies, pre-cut veggies, or your own home-prepared veggies into a quick meal in just minutes. You can use seasonings almost every time, except when you're cooking strong-flavored veggies such as onions, which need no further seasoning. Some thicker-leafed vegetables or roots take longer to tenderize; use low heat and simmer. Most will cook in a few minutes. Take turnip greens for instance, this deliciously aggressive-

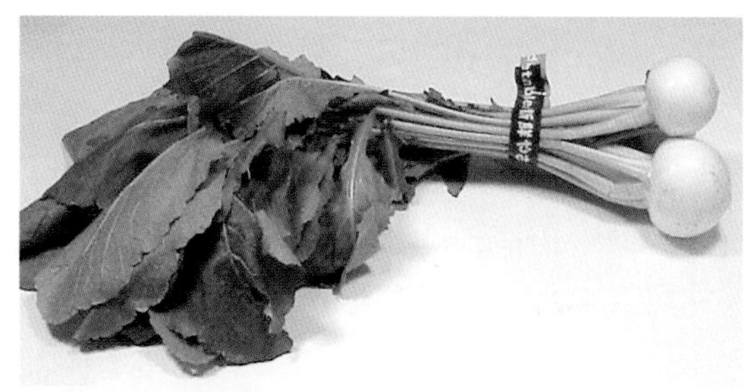

Tender turnip greens

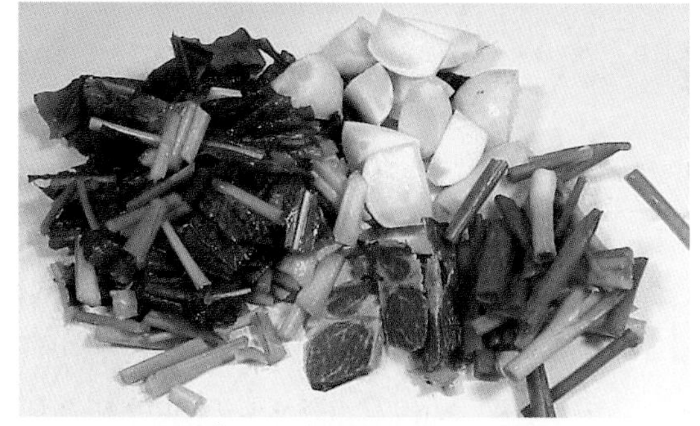

Cut greens, turnip, ham, and green onion

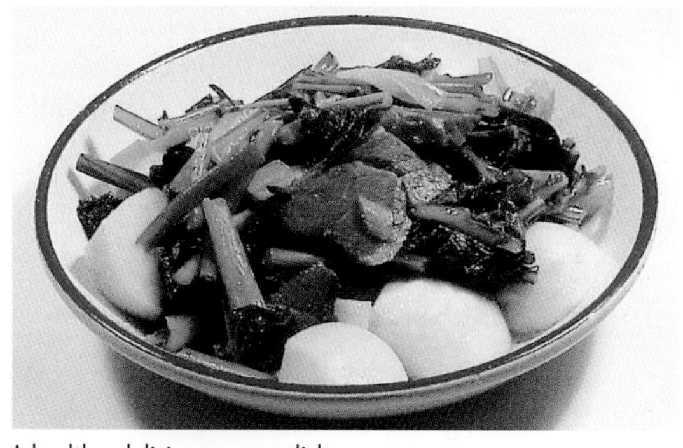

A healthy, delicious greens dish

tasting vegetable is very nutritious. The mature leaf is coarse and pungent, not very agreeable to most palates. Generally, we eat the root only, but young turnips with the green leaves are very popular among Japanese; they call it *Kabu.*

Just quarter the small turnips with the skins on, cut the leaves into one-inch or two-inch lengths, and simmer with whole garlic, ham, bacon, or any leftover meats. Simmered for ten minutes, it is delicious. You need to have your own turnip patch, though, or access to a Japanese market because that's the only place you can get young turnips. Older leaves taste strong and have a coarser texture; they're not as tender and delicious as the young ones. This is just an example; you can cook any young tender greens such as radish or daikon greens the same way. Heavy green leaves contain very valuable nutrients.

When cooking for young children, go easy on the seasonings at first. Kids usually like their veggies plain and cooked tender. But do use the stir-fry technique to cook the veggies.

Stir-Frying Meat

Meat, by nature, is a good insulator, which means it takes time for heat to penetrate and cook through. A thick cut of meat needs to be cooked rare; otherwise, the surface of the meat is overcooked and becomes tough and chewy. On the other hand, thin-sliced meat that is stir-fried very quickly on high heat results in much more tender meat, and it's easier to season properly.

The following is an example of using basic stir-fry techniques to cook New York steaks:

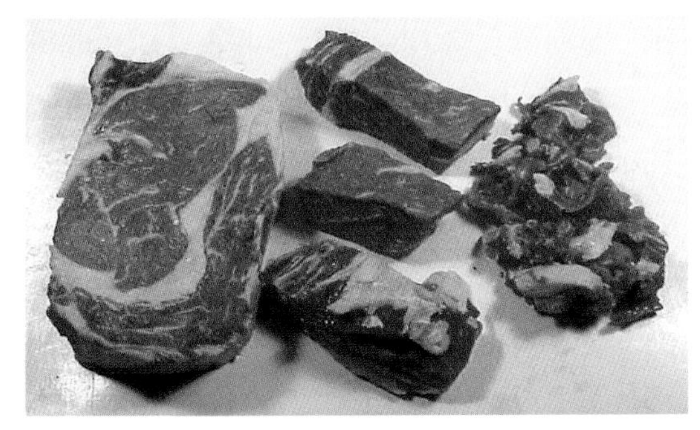

How to cut meat

1. Take a thick steak and cut it into one-inch strips; trim off excess fat. If you like your meat tender, soak it in a bowl of water with a teaspoon of baking soda for 30 minutes; then rinse thoroughly with clean water. Using a sharp knife, cut as thin as possible, vertically, against the grain of the meat.
2. Chop 3 to 4 stalks of green onions into half-inch sections.
3. Mix the following: 4 tablespoons teriyaki soy sauce, 2 tablespoons white wine, 2 tablespoons water, and $^1/_2$ teaspoon of sugar in a bowl. Optionally, you can add some jalapeño and black pepper.
4. Heat 2 to 3 tablespoons of olive oil in a heavy frying pan, 10 inches or larger if possible. Swirl the oil in the pan and heat until it begins to smoke.
5. Add the meat and onions, and stir until it starts to change color. It takes less than a minute.
6. Pour in your sauce and stir some more. Remove as soon as the sauce boils and the meat changes color. Cooking time depends on the thickness of the slices.

This dish is delicious, but as you can see, it contains only meat. You'll probably want to add vegetables to a meat dish like this. Vegetable enzymes tenderize the meat, and the overall dish ends up healthier.

The following example uses about one-half pound of thin sliced steak, one chopped onion, and jalapeños.

1. Thin-slice the meat and marinate with 2 tablespoonfuls each of teriyaki sauce, olive oil, and white wine for 30 minutes or more.

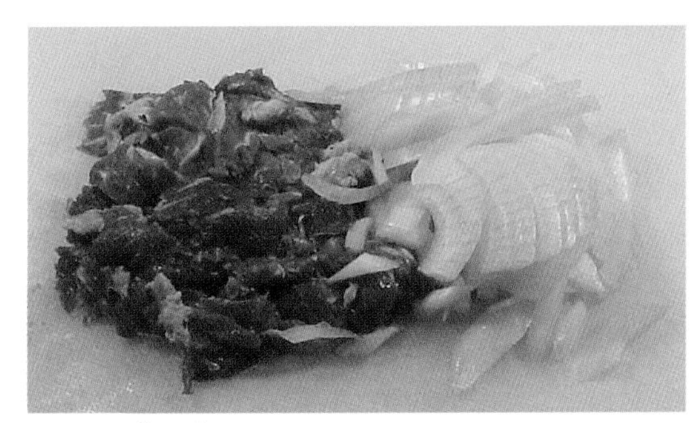

Getting it all ready

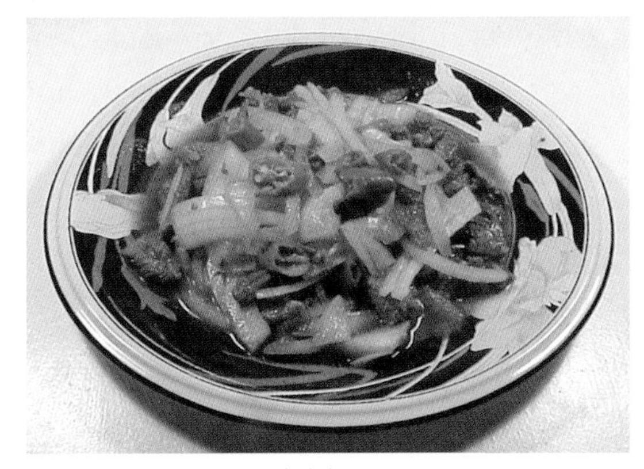

Simple, delicious onion steak dish

2. Place all ingredients in a very hot pan with olive oil, and stir quickly so the contents mix evenly.
3. Cover for 30 seconds; as soon as all of the meat turns a pale color, it is done.

This is a very delicious way to cook meat. Instead of the New York steak, you can substitute chicken, pork, lamb, or fish. Remember that fish cooks faster, so don't thin slice it; instead, cut it into pieces about one-half-inch thick. All meats taste good this way, and they will be tender because they are thin-sliced. Chopped onions also add flavor to meat, and they tenderize the meat as well. Even inexpensive meat tastes great when cooked this way.

Vegetables with Meat Dishes

You can use the same technique in two steps to make combination vegetable and meat dishes. Here's how to do it:

1. Stir-fry broccoli and set it aside on a plate.
2. Stir-fry New York steak. When the meat is cooked, add cooked broccoli, stir, and remove from heat immediately. This creates an instant, delicious beef broccoli dish. You can do the same with chicken, pork, veal, venison, or other meat.
3. Alternatively, pour the stir-fried New York steak over the broccoli plate so the meat will be on top of the broccoli.

This combination makes a delicious and attractive dish.

EXAMPLES OF STIR-FRIED READY-MIX SALAD GREENS

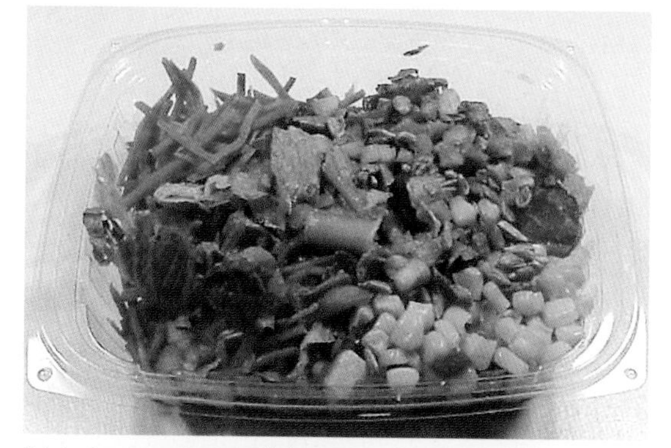

Original raw ready-mix salad greens

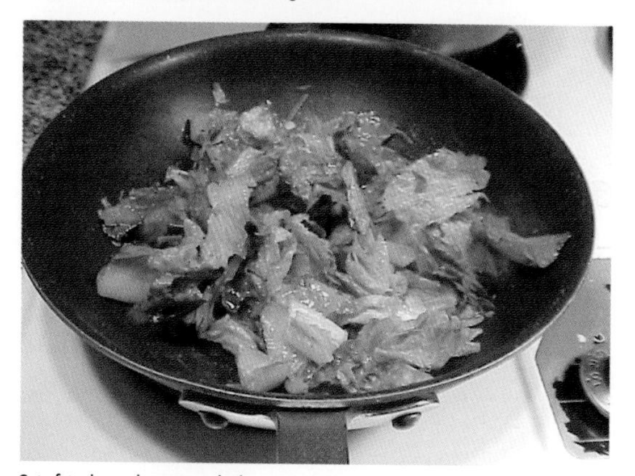

Stir-fried ready-mix salad

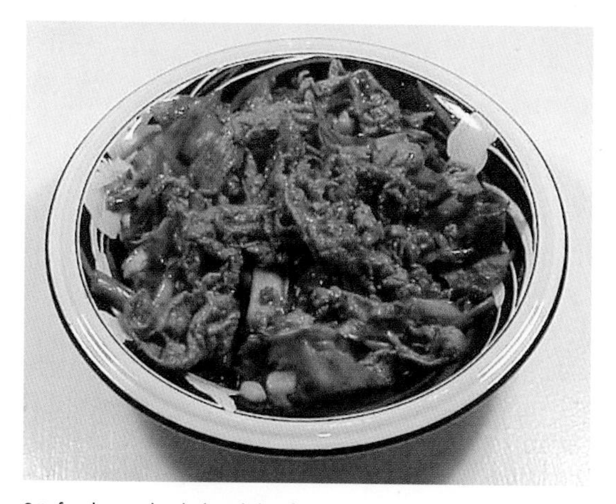

Stir-fried mixed salad with beef

The preceding photos showed an example of raw ready-mix salad vegetables from the market, one stir-fried, and one stir-fried with thin-sliced beef on top. This may be a new idea for you, but after you give it a try, I think you will like it. It is much healthier and more delicious than raw salad. This dish is wonderful served over steamed rice, as well. If you like fried rice, you will love the taste of this dish served over steamed rice.

You can stir-fry almost any vegetable: onions, green peppers, cabbage, green beans, squash, spinach, tomatoes, carrots, and so on. Using different combinations of vegetables and meats, hundreds of dishes can be created limited only by your imagination. For vegetarian dishes, substitute tofu, nuts, beans, or any food with high protein content for the meat.

More Ways to Cook Meat

Here's another method for cooking meat. In this example, I'm using New York steak strip.

1. Take a regular cut New York steak, pan-fry at medium heat, and brown it about 5 to 10 minutes each side to rare making sure not to overcook it.
2. Remove and cut into one-quarter-inch to three-eighths-inch strips.
3. Stir-fry with green onions and the teriyaki meat sauce mixture described above until done.
4. Alternatively, the meat can be cut and marinated with a tablespoon of olive oil, 1 to 2 tablespoons of teriyaki sauce, 1/2 teaspoon of sugar, one egg white, some wine, chopped garlic, or green onion, etc. Mix well, and let it sit in the refrigerator for at least 30 minutes.
5. Heat a pan to sizzling, add meat, stir-fry, turn heat to medium, and let cook for a minute or so. Since the meat is thick, it will take slightly longer than thin-sliced meat.
6. As soon as the meat changes color, cook 10 to 20 seconds more. The marinated mixture tenderizes the meat, and the mild ingredients will not alter or overpower the taste of the meat.

This is another delicious dish to eat, as is, or used to create more dishes.

By thin-slicing the steak or cutting meat into smaller pieces, we end up with a much more tender product, and we also end up eating less meat because of the greater bulk created by slicing the beef thin. Eating less meat may be important to overall good health.

Chunky Meat

Cornish Game Hen. I like Cornish game hens because they are smaller than

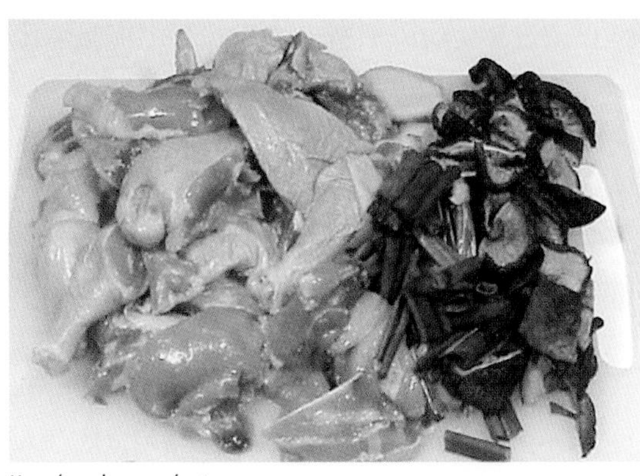

Hen/mushroom/onion

regular chickens and have less fat; however, any chicken or chicken part can be used.

1. Cut a Cornish game hen into pieces; you'll probably end up with legs, thighs, wings, and about four pieces of breast meat. Remove excess fat or skin.
2. In a bowl, add 1/2 cup of teriyaki sauce, 1/4 cup of sherry wine, 2 teaspoons of sugar, optional jalapeño, chili pepper, and vinegar.
3. Using a large, deep sauté pan, heat oil over high heat, sauté 5 to 6 slices of gingerroot, then add chicken and sauce. Sesame oil adds more flavor or yang to this dish.
4. The meat will release some moisture; let it simmer for a few minutes, and then adjust the sauce level to cover about two-thirds of the hen.
5. Cook over low heat, covered, for 20 to 30 minutes, longer if you like tender meat. Make sure to adjust the heat to low, since at high heat you can quickly dry out the sauce and char the meat.
6. Add green onions, cut 2 to 3 inches long, 5 minutes before serving.

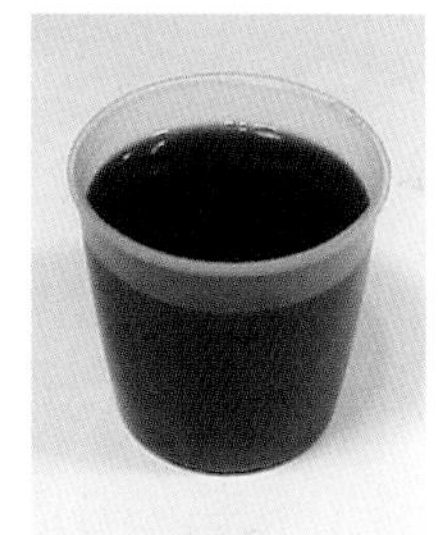

Sauce from cooking

You should have about one-half cup of sauce at the end of cooking. You can pour the sauce over rice for a delicious meal. Serve with stir-fried veggies alongside. This is a wonderful way to cook chicken wings. They make a fantastic appetizer.

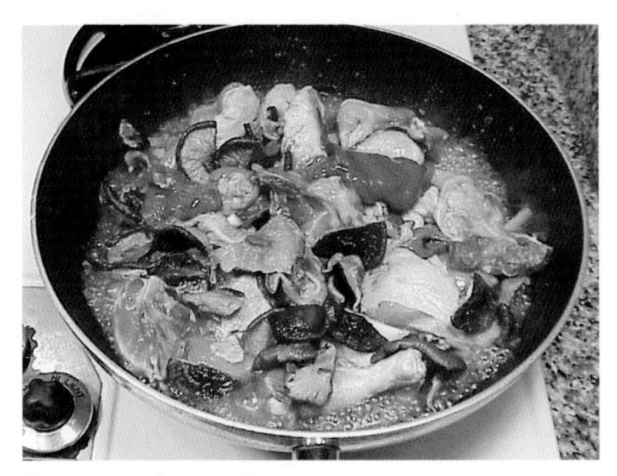

Mix, cover, and start cooking

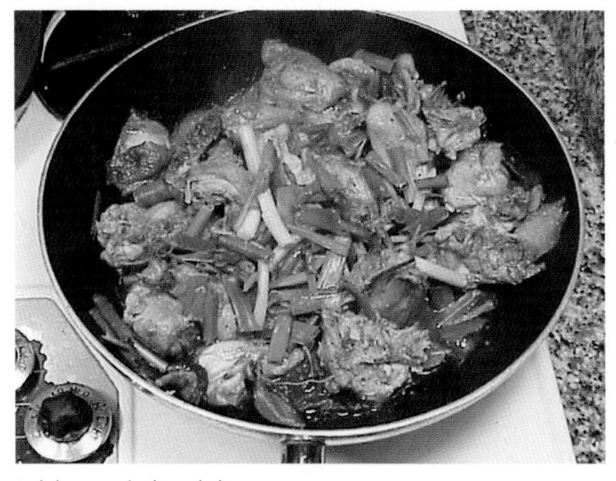

A delicious chicken dish

Soy Sauce Stew Dishes

This is a popular dish in Taiwan. The tender, stewed meat is covered with a delicious sauce at the end of cooking. You can pour the sauce over steamed rice and serve alongside the meat, the same as the Cornish game hen. Serve stir-fried vegetables with this sauce, as well. When I was growing up, we sometimes had only poor-quality rice cooked with dried sweet potatoes. It tasted pretty bad. This stewed meat with sauce produced a good meal in spite of the rice and dried sweet potatoes.

Make this dish with pork or beef, not too lean. You need some marbling for a moist, finished dish.

1. Cut meat into about 1-inch pieces. Trim off any excess fat, but leave some on. Alternatively, the meat may be cut into larger chunks, perhaps into two-by-four-inch pieces. You can end up eating more meat, but larger pieces of meat retain more moisture.
2. Mash peeled ginger and other seasonings you might like. Bay leaf and thyme are great stewed this way. For a special Chinese flavor, add a tablespoon of star anise seed.
3. Add a teaspoon of whole peppercorns, 1/4 to 1/2 cup of teriyaki sauce, 1/4 cup of water, and a scant teaspoon of sugar.
4. Add 1/2 cup of either red wine, white wine, whisky, or brandy. The alcohol content will boil off leaving a rich dimension to the sauce. Remember that the color of red wine will change the color of the dish. White wine, sake, or rice wine is better to maintain a light color. Most red wines add a dark, soy sauce-like color.
5. Adjust the water level until the sauce almost covers the meat. Bring to a boil and simmer for about 45 minutes. Simmer only; the heat needs to be as low as possible. High heat will not cook it any faster; it simply evaporates out the sauce more quickly, and fast cooked meats are drier than slow cooked meats.
6. Five minutes before serving, cut three to four green onions into 2-inch pieces and add to the stewed meat. Be sure to remove the ginger, anise seed, and peppercorns before serving.

Root vegetables such as daikon and carrots are often stewed with meat this way, and the enzymes from these roots tenderize the meat and add special flavor. Daikon, in particular, tastes good and is very popular.

Try this daikon-meat dish. Peel and cut the daikon radish into half-inch cubes to cook with the meat as above; use equal amounts of daikon and meat making sure the sauce covers the meat and the daikon.

You can add chopped onions or green onions, as well. The radish takes about the same amount of time to stew as the meat. The flavors of the meat and daikon blend well, but we end up eating less meat, and we get the benefit of the complex enzymes in the radish and the onions, as well. If daikon is not available, use carrots. This dish tastes delicious made with any good cut of beef or lamb.

Although it is fine to do this on the stove, this dish cooks particularly nice in a Crockpot. You can start it in the morning, set it to low, and have a perfectly cooked meat dish when you get home from work. You may need to reduce liquid content with a Crockpot since much less liquid will evaporate. (There are more details in the following section).

If you like, twenty minutes before serving, you can add cubed tofu to this dish. The flavor of the sauce will permeate the tofu. If you use tofu this way, you will enjoy the health benefits and stretch the meat needed for a meal. When I was growing up, my mother used this technique to make a large meal with only one-half pound of pork.

How to Cook Spare Ribs

Most Americans barbecue spare ribs, which can turn out tough and hard to eat. However, you can stew spare ribs the same as you did the pork and beef above, and it turns into a delightful dish. Pork ribs, especially baby spare ribs, are very good prepared this way. When you stew spare ribs, the sauce picks up the minerals in the bones so it's a natural source of calcium and other minerals.

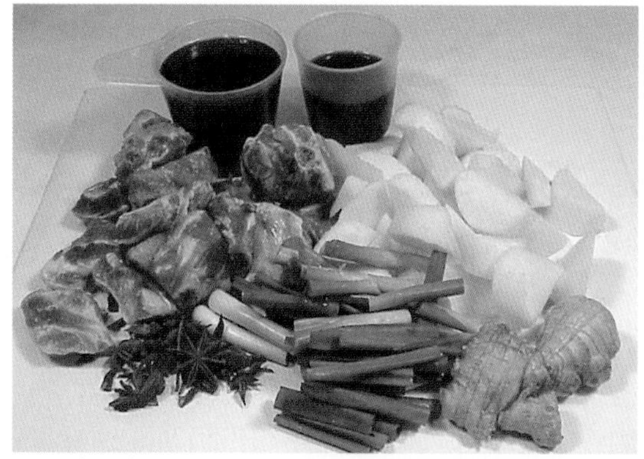

Cut and ready.

Buy about two pounds of spare ribs and have the butcher make two cuts, sawing the meat so that each rib is in three sections, each section about two to three inches long. Separate each rib to make about one-by-two-inch to one-by-three-inch pieces.

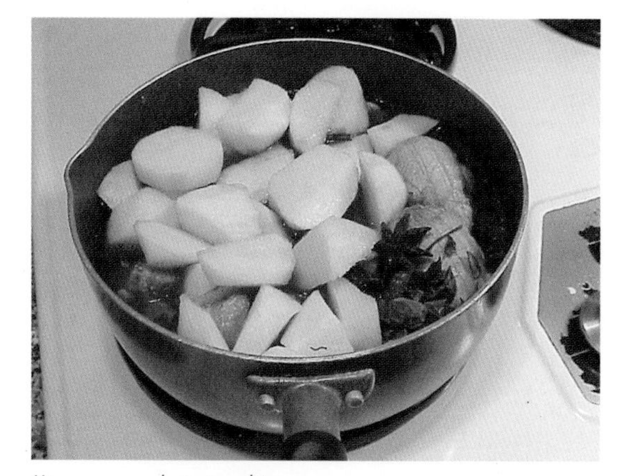

Mix, cover, and start cooking.

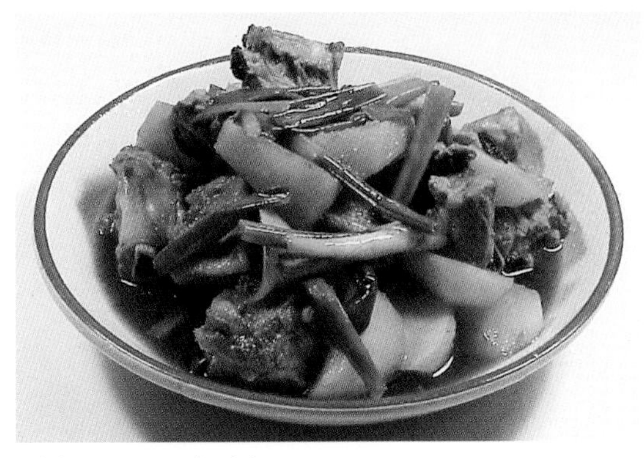

A delicious spare ribs dish

Cook as above. Again, daikon is the most popular vegetable to stew this way; it makes the ribs much more tender. You can also cook the meat in one piece, uncut, for about an hour. After the ribs are done, you can slice them into serving portions and place on a plate topped with the sauce.

This type of dish is very easy to cook in a large quantity; after cooking, divide it into meal portions, and freeze it. The ribs are easily warmed later by placing them in a steamer to cook with rice. You could also use the microwave oven.

Use Your Automatic Rice Cooker to Cook Meats

With an automatic rice cooker, you add rice and the correct amount of water according to the marks on the pot. After the cooking cycle, the rice is cooked, and the water has boiled away. When this happens, the temperature of the cooker increases rapidly, and a thermostat switches the cooker to the 'keep-warm mode.' During the keep-warm mode, lower heat is supplied to keep the rice warm until the cooker is unplugged. The temperature of the rice drops slowly over a few hours from the water's boiling temperature of 212°F to about 150°F where it stays. Knowing how the cooker works, we can use it to cook other dishes. Slow-cooked meat and veggies cooked in the rice cooker generally taste juicy and moist.

Another Way to Slow-Cook Meat

Take a mixing bowl with no handles (about six cups capacity or larger), one that will fit into your rice cooker with the cover on. Put the meat and other ingredients to be stewed inside the bowl. Place about one-half to one cup of water inside the cooker and set the bowl, with the food in the bowl, inside the cooker. Now, start the cooker in the morning. The cooker will start to boil in a few minutes and continue about thirty minutes; that will also bring the contents of the mixing bowl to a boil.

When the cooker switches to keep-warm mode, the meat and veggies will not be cooked yet. As the cooker stays in keep-warm mode, however, they continue to cook until dinnertime. They end up tasting great when cooked slowly like this.

The amount of water inside the cooker determines the boiling time, which depends on the kind of meat. To cook a couple of pounds of spare ribs, for instance, a cup of water works best since pork takes longer to cook, while one-half cup of water is better for a two pound chicken. This way, the meat is boiled for about twenty minutes and continues to cook slowly as the temperature comes down to 150°F. Alternatively, you can place enough water in the cooker to boil for a desired period of time, and then manually switch to "keep warm" mode.

Use carrots or daikon to cook with meat and the resulting dish will be extra juicy, moist, and tender. Be aware, though, that veggies cooked this way must be able to withstand the long cooking time, so stick to onions, carrots, and Daikon.

Place ingredients inside a mixing bowl, put one cup of water inside the cooker, then place the mixing bowl inside the cooker. Plug the cooker in and start cooking.

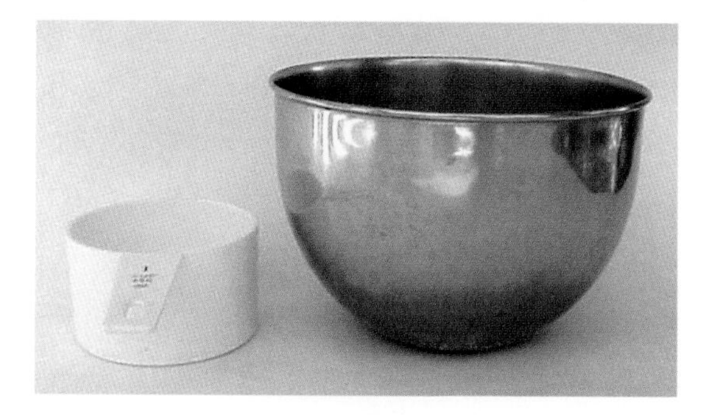

Crockpot or Slow Cooker

The slow cooker operates differently from the rice cooker. The slow cooker applies low heat constantly. It takes time for the contents to come to a boil, and the food continues to gently boil until the Crockpot is turned off, while the rice cooker brings the temperature to a boil quickly for a short time, and then slowly cools down. Both are good to stew meat unattended, but meat and veggies taste slightly different.

The Rice Cooker As a Steamer

Most automatic rice cookers come with one or two steamer inserts designed to sit in the upper part of the cooker. If you put the veggies in at the same time as you start the rice, most of them will end up overcooked since veggies steam quickly. You can add the veggies to the steamer halfway through cooking the rice. Leftover meat or other leftovers that can withstand steaming for a longer time are a different story. You can add these foods at the same time as the rice and end up with dinner ready for very little effort. If you want to use the rice cooker as a steamer, just place the food in the steamer, add water, turn on the rice cooker, and then unplug it when the food is done.

Meatballs

This is somewhat similar to making meat loaf except it's cooked differently.

1. Chop one onion into about one-quarter-inch pieces.
2. In a mixing bowl, place about 1 pound of hamburger meat.
3. Add a chopped onion, 2 egg whites, 1/4 cup of olive oil, 1/4 cup of white wine, 1/4 cup of teriyaki soy sauce, and 2 to 3 tablespoons of cornstarch.
4. Salt, pepper, and herbs to taste. You can also add Mexicorn or cooked rice to stretch the meat. Garlic powder, oregano, and thyme taste good in meatballs as well, in small amounts, and you can also add a dash of chili powder.
5. Shape meatballs into 1- or 2-inch balls.
6. Make a teriyaki sauce as described earlier, bring it to a boil, then reduce the heat to medium.
7. Place the meatballs, one at a time, into the boiling sauce.
8. Simmer the whole batch over low heat for 10 to 20 minutes.

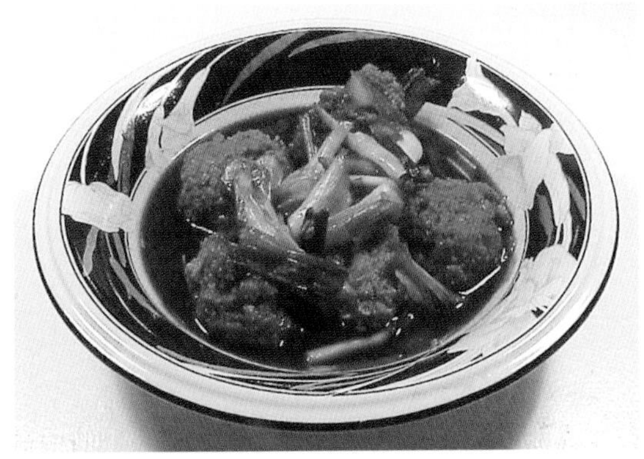

Meatball dish

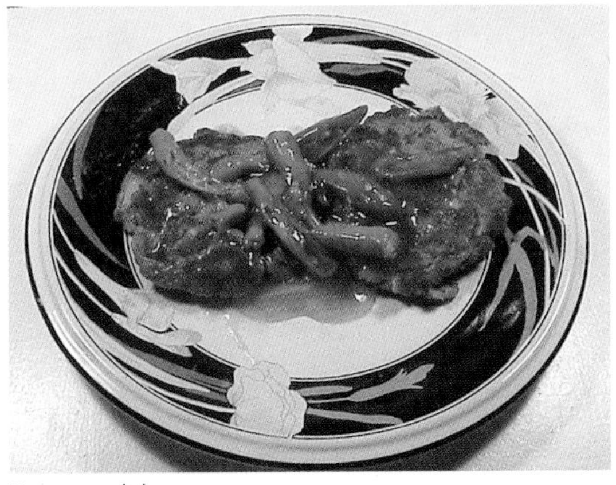

Meat patty dish

These are great cooked with daikon or carrots, but be sure to cut the veggies quite thin since the cooking time is short.

Curry Mix, a Tasty Meal

You can choose from many pre-mixed sauces that you can add with fresh ingredients to make a healthy and tasty dish. My favorite is Vermont Curry Mix, which has a mild and rich taste. The recipe requires about one to two pounds of meat or a Cornish hen, one onion, one potato, and 1 to 2 cups of carrots.

Cut all ingredients into bite size. Sauté with a couple tablespoons of olive oil, then add water to cover, and let simmer with the cover on for 20 minutes, or until the ingredients

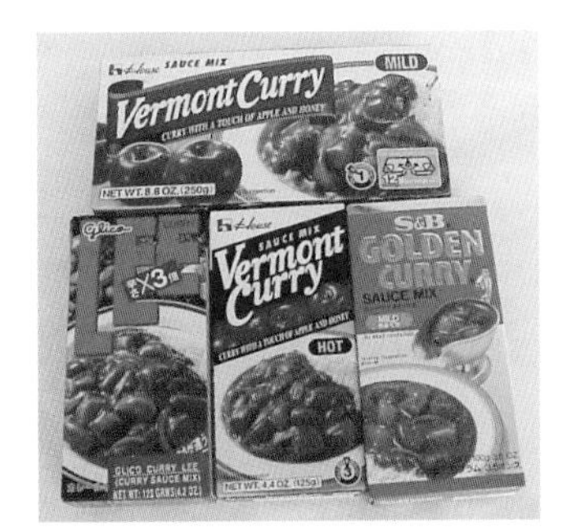

are tender. Add curry mix at low heat, and stir until the sauce mix melts and the sauce thickens.

This is a wonderful dish to serve over rice or noodles. There are many types of curry mixes from mild and gently sweet to red-hot. Read the label carefully. Curry is a healthy food for the heart and digestive system.

Seafood

As you may already know, Taiwan is an island and we love seafood. Most of our dishes would not be practical to include here; however, I have added some simple, basic ones.

Stir-Fried Shrimp

Take about one-half pound to one pound of shrimp with shells and heads removed. Medium-size shrimp are better for this dish; if you have large tiger shrimp, slice them open lengthwise from the bottom side. It is good to soak them in milk for a while to remove any chemical odors since chemicals are often used as a preservative.

Mix together about two tablespoons of teriyaki sauce, two tablespoons of sherry wine, and two egg whites; be sure to mix them well. Heat the pan at high heat with olive oil, add green onions and shrimp, stir

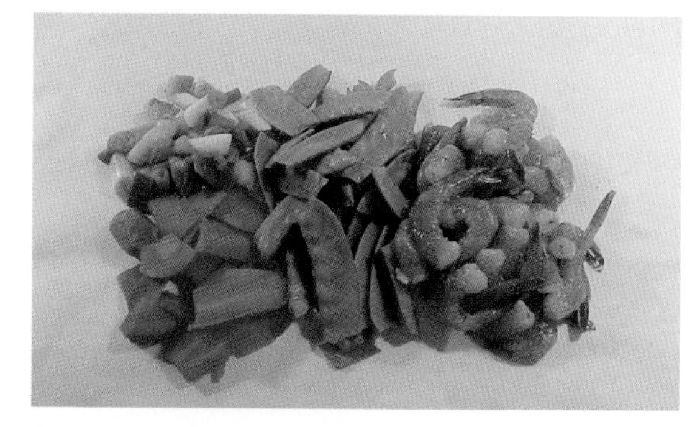

Carrot, green onion, snow pea and shrimp

a few times, add the sauce mix, and quickly reduce heat to medium-low. Let the sauce boil for a few seconds.

As soon as the shrimp changes color evenly, it is done. Shrimp cooked correctly should be crunchy and sweet. Overcooked shrimp can be hard and chewy, and their flavor deteriorates badly.

To add vegetables to this shrimp dish, it is easier to stir-fry veggies separately. Prepare veggies as described earlier, and then add the finished shrimp, and heat for a few seconds; do not overcook. It is popular to prepare shrimp with snow peas, Napa cabbage, or regular cabbage.

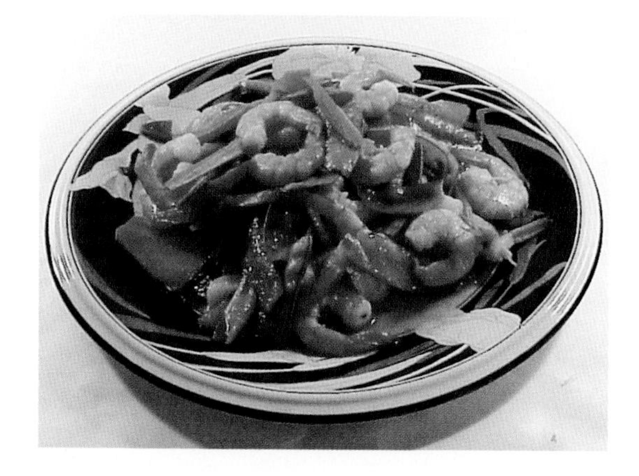

Pan-Fried Fish Steak

Asians like smaller fish such as sea bass, mackerel, and sea trout. These fish usually weigh no more than three pounds and the cooked meat is sweet and moist. Pan-frying is the usual method used by Asians to cook fish. Here is how they do it:

1. Heat 1 to 2 tablespoons of olive oil in a non-stick pan.
2. Using medium heat, place the fish in the pan and move them around to make sure the fish are coated with oil and will not stick to the pan.
3. Cook a few minutes until brown and turn over.
4. Cover to steam and brown at the same time; when cooking is finished, there should not be any moisture left. If necessary, remove cover and increase heat to evaporate any moisture.
5. Season with salt and pepper, or add a couple spoonfuls of a teriyaki sauce and wine mixture.
6. Cover and let simmer a minute, and then remove immediately. Alternatively, pan-fried fish can be removed onto a plate without seasoning.
7. Chop 3 to 4 tablespoons of scallion, stir-fry with olive oil, and add seasoning of teriyaki sauce and wine mixture.
8. Remove as soon as the sauce starts to boil, and then pour over the fish on the plate.

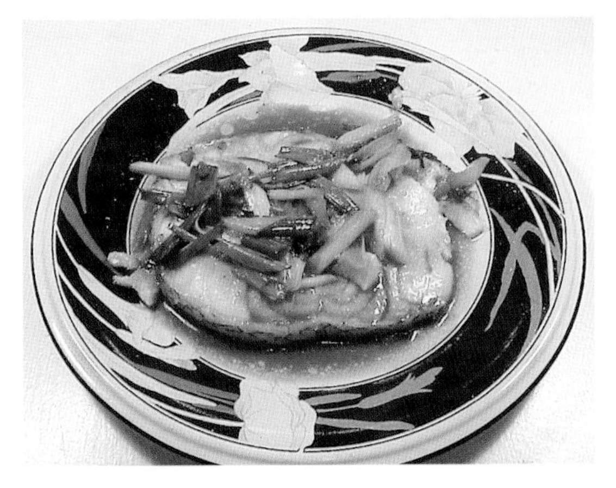

Fish such as sea trout and Chilean sea bass can take quite a bit of cooking; after such cooking, the meat tastes sweet and tender.

Chilean Sea Bass Dish

The difficult fish are salmon, shrimp, and trout because when they are overcooked, they are dry and lose much of their flavor. To retain as much moisture within the flesh as possible, depending on the thickness of the fish, let it fry for about three minutes on each side until brown, but still red or pink in the middle. Cover the pan, turn off the heat, and let it sit for five to ten minutes. It tastes best when the middle part is slightly pinkish or a little red along the center bone of the trout or salmon.

Steaming is the best way to cook fresh fish. Season the fish and place in a steamer for about seven minutes. Fresh seafood doesn't need much seasoning.

Good seafood has a natural, sweet taste and flavor. Any seasoning can easily overwhelm the natural taste of seafood. For example, in Chinese cookery, the most popular way to cook live shrimp is to steam them quickly; as soon as the shrimp shells change color, remove from heat. The shrimp is peeled and dipped into a very light sauce. The only taste you get is the fresh, sweet shrimp taste.

Seafood is at its best when just caught, right from the ocean. Even live fish, crabs, and lobsters in the aquariums at restaurants lose muscle and don't taste as good, the longer they are kept after capture. Seafood that is not fresh needs to be deep fried or heavily seasoned to cover its strong taste.

'Join the Devil'

Reading this book, it sounds easy to cook fresh everyday. I think most of us wish that we could. Yet even if we made a total commitment to stay away from processed foods, I doubt we could really do it, especially if youngsters are involved. We might as well agree to eat processed foods once in awhile because these are the foods your family likes now, but we can do it with a twist of common sense. Here are some ideas to try:

Meat Stew. You can buy canned or frozen meat stews everywhere. Just stir-fry some veggies and add them to the stew. You can add leftover rice or a can of corn, as well; both have a neutral taste and blend well with stew meat. This will stretch the product and give you healthier meals, as well.

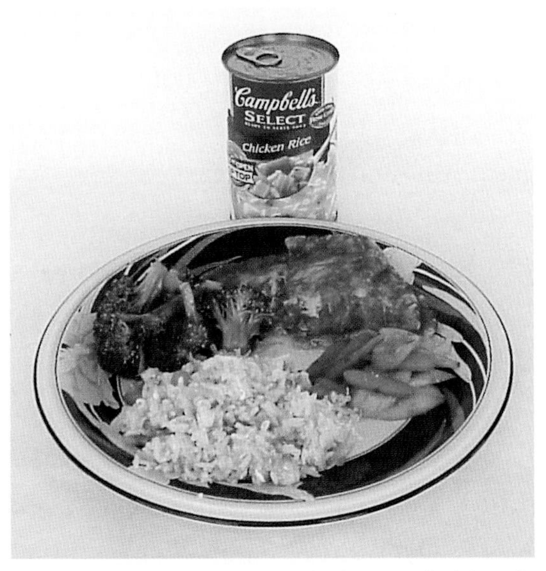

An example of a pizza dinner with fried rice, stir-fried broccoli, marinated veggies, and canned soup.

Canned Soup. Again, stir-fry some chopped veggies or add tofu or corn to the soup. The idea is to add fresh nutrients to the processed food.

Hamburgers, Pizza, and Similar 'Junk' Food. Instead of having junk food as the entire meal, stir-fry some veggies and serve them alongside the other food. Slice hamburgers into four portions and eat the portions as *part* of the meal. Stir-fry a couple of dishes to make up the rest. The rule is to eat your veggies first before the junk food. If you make a bowl of vegetable soup to eat with hamburgers or pizza, you'll be surprised at how good a meal it is, and it can be healthy too.

Plan ahead, keep going, and add healthy vegetable dishes to your meals everyday. If you persist, you can change your family's diet in a fairly short time.

As you have seen, the cooking techniques here are very simple and flexible. You'll find it easier to create meals if you begin to take this approach. I've suggested certain ingredients, but you can use any vegetables and meats that you like. The goal is to have a diet with many different kinds of foods prepared fresh each day. Once you master these techniques, you can enjoy a variety of wonderful dishes, which are always new and interesting.

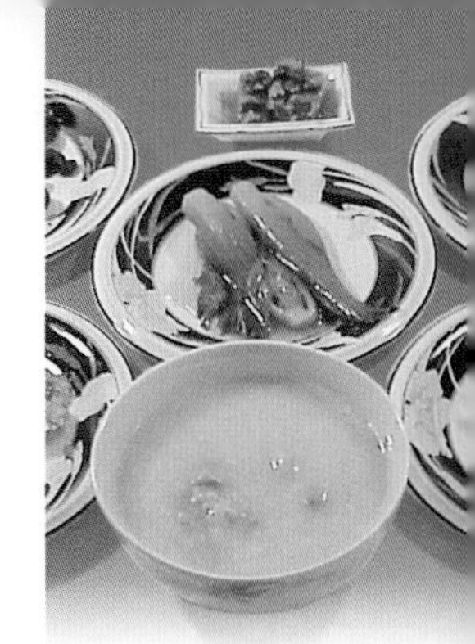

Chapter 11

Stocks, Soups, and Porridges

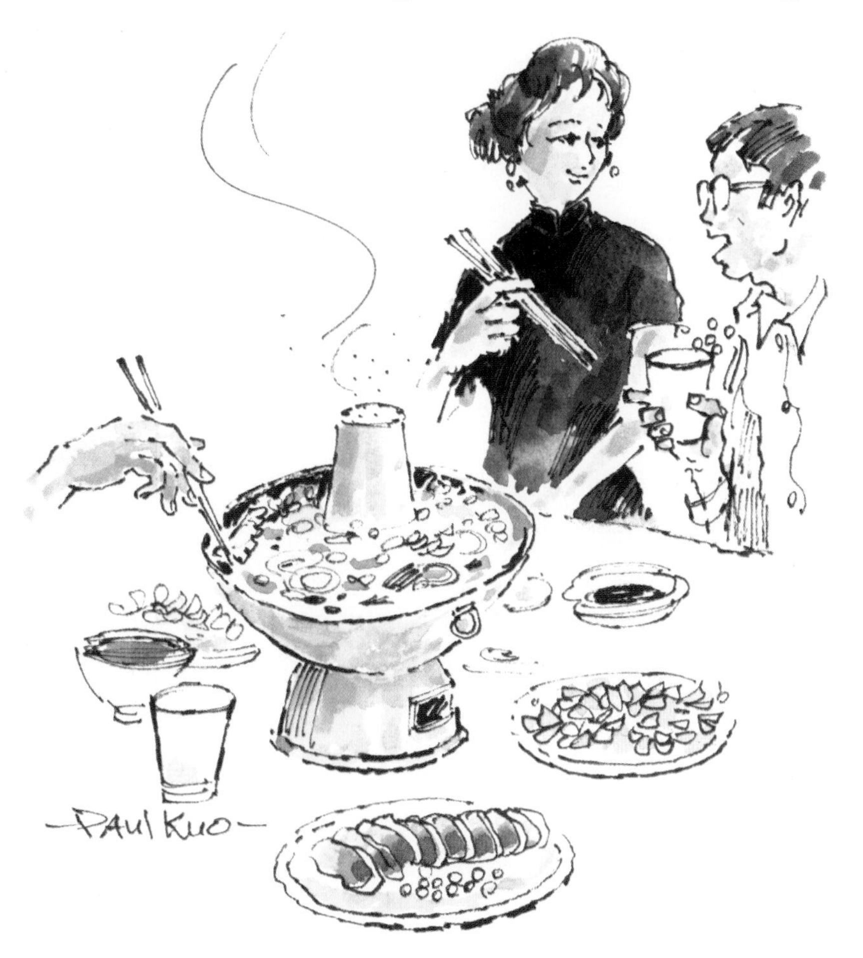

By now, we can see that the only way to have a good diet is to get in there and create it for ourselves. Soup and porridge are both vital to a first-rate diet, but you can't buy the quality you can make at home cheaply and easily. Both foods can go a long way to create excellent health, but unfortunately, most of us don't use them much in our everyday nutrition. And probably the only way we eat porridge is as a sweetened breakfast cereal. Yet porridge can be a major solution for many of our modern health problems.

In most international cuisines, fresh homemade soup is a common starter for the main meal, and porridges have been eaten with meats and vegetables for ages in various parts of the world. They are both very satisfying and nutritious but not fattening. In many large cities in Asia, you can even find porridge restaurants to serve those who want to eat light and bland. Porridge restaurants serve simple rice porridge with vegetables and pickles only. Recently, this kind of food has gained popularity as the standard of living has improved, and people have become more aware of the problems that come from overeating.

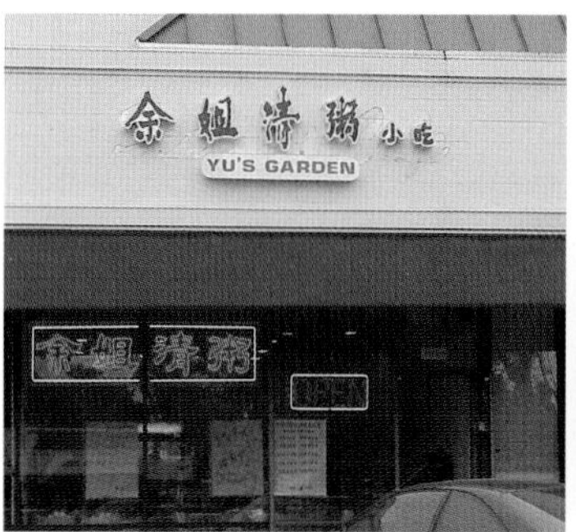

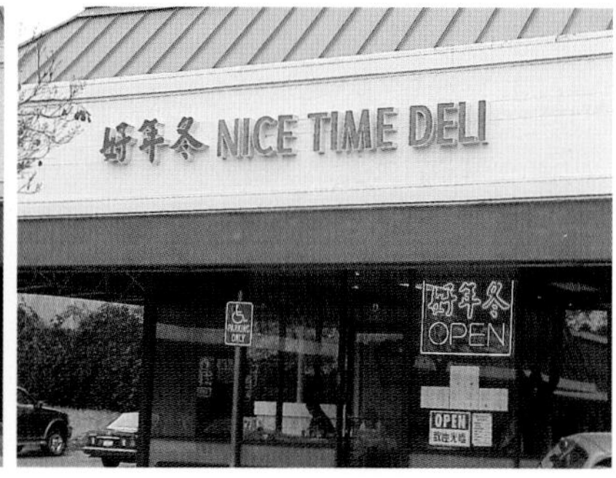

Chinese characters in neon signs say 'Light Porridge' and the menu is posted on the window.

In America, most Chinatowns have porridge restaurants; typically small restaurants that don't even bother to advertise or use English signage because they don't expect to serve American customers. It is difficult to find such restaurants if you can't read Chinese. Many large Chinese restaurants serve porridges also, especially during the weekend, but these foods are offered on special menus and only in Chinese.

There is no real fast-food alternative for first-rate soup and porridge; we have to make them. Stock is an excellent starting point for making wholesome porridge, as well as soup.

How to Make Stock

You can make good stock many different ways, but the standard procedure is to use beef bones, chicken bones, or a whole chicken, and simmer in plenty of water in a stockpot for three to four hours or all day in a Crockpot. Boil the bones or chicken for ten minutes first, then discard the water and rinse the bones, then add fresh water to start again. This gives you a clean, clear broth. Skim off any fat or foam floating on the surface periodically during cooking to keep the broth clear. You can add onions, celery, leeks, daikon, and carrots for flavor and nutrients.

Daikon and onions are very good for making stock. It's better to stay with these veggies and not experiment too much since strong-flavored vegetables can alter the flavor of the stock. When the stock is done, filter it through cheesecloth—and that's it. Don't add potatoes until you are ready to serve since they thicken and cloud the stock. Make plenty of stock so you can freeze some for future use.

Animal bones are rich in minerals and other nutrients including some rare compounds. Stocks contain collagen, which helps our body absorb water. You can reheat it and cook it again; it can be stored in the fridge for about three days or frozen for longer. It will often become jelled when cold. This indicates that you have a good, rich broth. Don't salt until you're ready to use the stock.

To flavor your stock, try adding mashed garlic or mashed ginger, peppercorns, bay leaves, basil, and oregano. For beef or lamb stock, try some rosemary. For example, for two quarts of stock add two cloves of garlic, one to two teaspoons of mashed ginger, one-quarter to one-half teaspoon of peppercorns, one to two bay leaves, and/or one-half to one teaspoon each of basil and oregano.

You can make quantities of stock over the weekend, divide it into portions and pour into freezer bags, and then save it in the freezer. If you prepare a lot of stock once a month and use it throughout the month, you might not need calcium supplements. Properly made broth or stock can provide plenty of calcium in the natural balance we need. A good stock can be the basis for an excellent soup and is often used in non-breakfast porridges.

Soups

In most traditional cultures, soup is a very important part of the meal. A bowl of

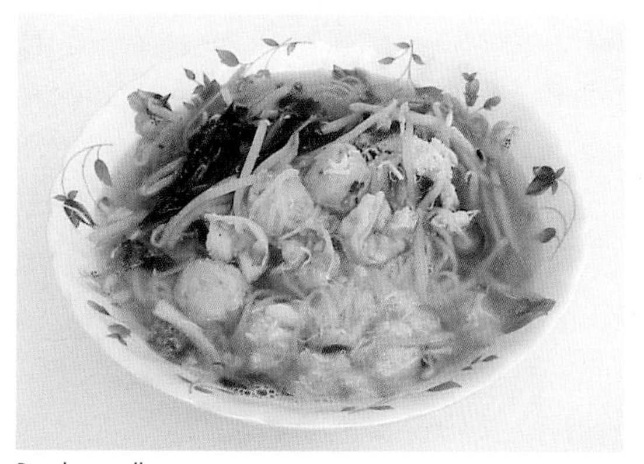

Popular noodle soup

warm soup is comforting and, at the same time, it supplies healthy nutrients, which are easy to digest and absorb. Served with bread or other similar foods, soup is filling and satisfying. It can help heavier, drier foods 'go down' more easily. Recent research has shown that people who eat soup everyday lose weight more consistently.

While most of us don't eat soup with most meals anymore, we use something else to supply liquid to the meal like soft drinks. Can you imagine eating a hamburger, pizza, french fries, or a sandwich without a soda? We drink soft drinks copiously and then wonder why we're having health problems. Lots of our favorite fast foods are crisp, dry, and difficult to eat without washing them down with something.

Traditionally, soups were clear, light broths specifically made to help 'wash food down' and aid in digestion. Now we seem to have no choice but to drink icy cold soft drinks; we rarely ever see clear soups anymore. Today our soups are very heavy, thick, and creamy such as clam chowder, creamy broccoli, and potato soups. These soups are loaded with butter, cream or milk, and similar ingredients, which are too rich to be healthy. Clear soup, or broth when offered, is mostly over seasoned, very salty, and not very popular today.

A Quick, Healthy Soup

You can easily make this broth by sautéing green onions or shallots the same as you do stir-fry and sometimes adding bacon or ham to enhance the flavor. In a large stew pot, add an appropriate amount of liquid and let it boil; then add vegetables and tofu; for example, spinach, Napa cabbage, regular cabbage, cucumber, and/or thin-sliced or shredded carrots are all popular home-style soup ingredients. Season the soup with salt, pepper, and a little MSG, and it is light and bland. Liquid for the soup can be just water, pure soup stock, or any mixture of the two. Strong flavored or salty soups can cause excessive thirst; most people agree that it's better to avoid excess salt.

Another way to make soup is to boil a few sections of spare ribs and a few slices of Virginia ham for about thirty minutes at very low heat. When you cook it on low heat, you don't have to pay any attention to it, and the food will taste better too. Add carrots, onions, turnips, or thin sliced daikon and cook until tender. This soup is wonderful and loaded with mineral nutrients from the rib bones.

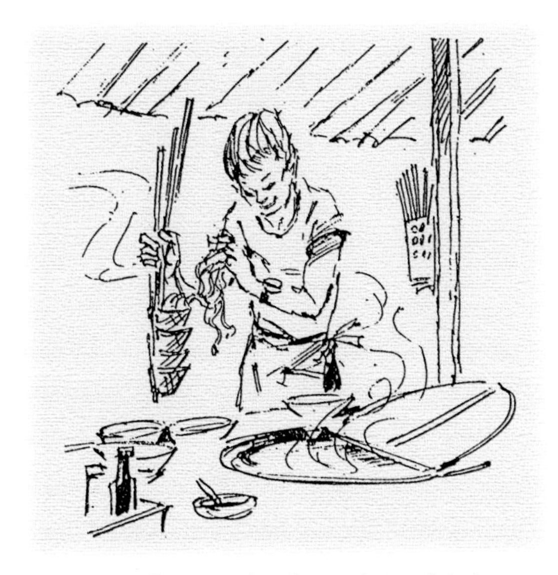

Minute noodles. A swish and a swash through boiling water suffices to cook these thin noodles. Soy sauce, pepper, and a dash of oil complete the dish.

Chicken Soup

Place a Cornish game hen in a mixing bowl and cover with water. The bowl should be big enough to hold the meat and the veggies, yet small enough to place in your rice cooker and be covered properly. Add daikon or carrots (veggies that can stand long cooking) and season to taste. Do not over salt; it is easier to add additional salt after cooking. Place the bowl inside the rice cooker, add one cup of water to start the steaming process, and then when it turns from 'cook' to 'warm,' let it sit for a few hours. The rice cooker automatically stays warm, and you will end up with a great chicken soup.

If you enjoy ginseng or dong quai, place a few pieces of Wisconsin ginseng or some dong quai in the pot to cook with the soup. If you use the herbs, it is better not to use veggies; instead, use a piece of mashed gingerroot. Ginseng and dong quai can break up after long simmering, so place them inside a small tea strainer or piece of cheesecloth. Peppercorns added to these herbs will also create a good flavor.

Ready-Mix Soup Base

There are many types of ready-mix soups available such as sweet and sour soup

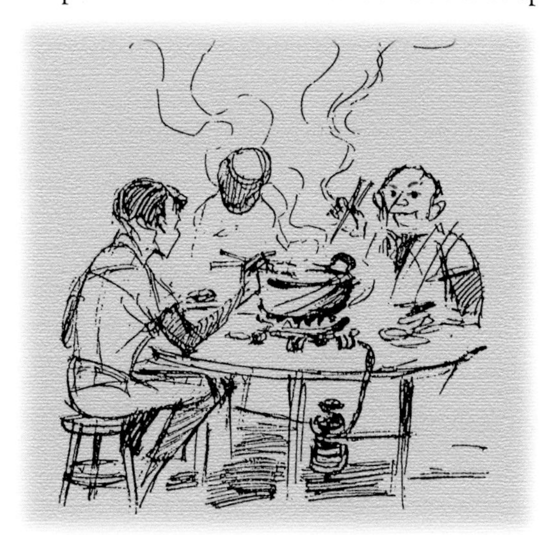

Around the steaming pot. Swatow beef is recommended for those who want something new. This cold weather dish consists of paper thin slices of beef cooked for an instant in boiling herbs. The bite of beef is bathed in pepper sauce and inhaled. "Water!"

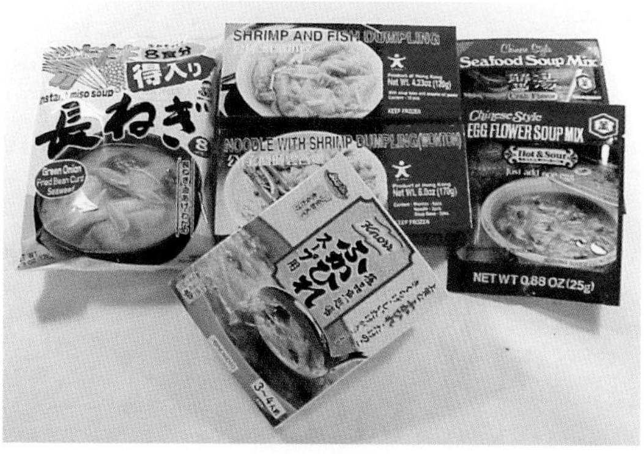

Ready-to-use soup mix, all you need to do is add veggies or eggs.

mix or egg flour soup mix; all you need to do is add eggs and/or vegetables. Use more water than the packages call for and always add fresh vegetables. In Japanese markets, there are many types of ready-mix bases for cooking, as well as for making soup.

One popular brand is made of bonito fish, while others use squid. The bonito fish or squid stock processed with salt and other ingredients, then made into granules, is a very popular form of soup base available in these markets. The broth base does not taste fishy but retains the savory taste of glutamate, which makes an excellent soup base. It is easy to use, similar to using seasoned salts. The little seasoning bag, which accompanies instant noodles, usually contains this broth mix.

Of course, some other additives come with the package, but that is the price you pay for convenience; however, the authentic home preparation from scratch is still the best way.

Porridge

Cereals are seeds of plants enclosed by a tough case for protection; these seeds are designed by nature to contain all the nutrients the baby plant will need. Grains are mostly made of starch, which will not dissolve in cold water, although they can absorb a certain amount of water when soaked. As grains are heated in water, they take in more liquid and finally burst, which releases starch into the water and thickens the mixture. Cereals cooked this way are digestible and nutritious, perhaps the ideal way to eat grains.

Historically, cereal porridges were often eaten by humble folk who could not afford much high-protein food, and who found the soft, warm cereal comforting. It was an important dish for the military in early cultures, as well as a common breakfast for all classes, although the wealthier folk often added meat. All human cultures have relied on some form of porridge throughout the ages. There is no specific definition for porridge, although in this country, oatmeal, cream of wheat, and other hot cereals are commonly eaten with sugar in the morning.

The Taiwanese call porridge gruel, congee, or soupy rice. Theoretically, any grain cereal can be cooked into porridge with other foods added for variety. Just like stir-frying, once you try it and get familiar with the basic technique, you can cook many different variations of porridge.

The Benefits of Porridge

A cup of grain generally cooks into five to eight cups of porridge. Take brown rice, for example; one cup of brown rice can boil into six to ten cups of thick porridge. You can add vegetables or meats to enhance flavor and add more nutrients. This can turn into a nutritious, warm, hearty, balanced meal, which is totally satisfying with minimum calories. It is an ideal dish to complement our rich diet today, and excellent to lose weight fast or just maintain your ideal weight.

When we have a cold, we often find chicken soup comforting, and it seems to shorten the duration of the cold. We may not understand why this happens, but it is obvious that our body likes it. If we need to stretch a chicken to feed a crowd, chicken soup is a good solution. Porridge can also help to fight a cold. When I feel a cold coming on, I eat simple, plain porridge for a couple of days to give my body a break and allow it to fight the cold virus.

Basic Porridge

Making porridge is very easy; just boil grain in water until the grain bursts and the starch combines with the water to make a thick mixture. Here is how to cook rice porridge:

Start with cooked rice, which saves time. To a cup of cooked rice, add about four cups of water; use six cups of water for uncooked rice, and again, use brown rice instead of white rice if you are health conscious. Use a large pot because it can boil over easily. Bring to a boil, then reduce heat to as low as possible, and let it simmer for one-half hour to one hour. Check and stir occasionally and add water when necessary; how much water you need depends on the heat applied. When it's done, turn off the heat and let it stand until cool enough to eat. It gets thicker as it sits. You can add more broth or warm water to thin the porridge, as needed.

Most automatic rice cookers come with a special pot to cook soupy rice; actually any slow cooker will also do a good job. Again, remember it can boil over easily, especially when using higher heat. Think *slow* when you cook porridge.

Cooked porridge continues to absorb the water and gets thicker as time goes on. You'll need to add extra water if you want to reheat it in a pot or a microwave oven for later. Any cereal, beans, peas, and roots can be cooked this way.

Any unseasoned breakfast cereal can make porridge, such as oatmeal, wheat germ, cream of wheat, grits, etc. Plain, hot cereals are porridge and similar to soupy rice except each has their unique characteristic taste and texture. All can be made into fancy porridge like soupy rice. See below.

Gourmet Porridge Meal

Plain porridge is thick and basic, but don't bring out the sugar bowl, cream, and butter just yet. To get the best of porridge, we need to find some other ways to eat it. This may be very different from what you ate as a child, but I think you might like it. Here are some methods to prepare creative porridge dishes.

Simple, Plain Porridge

Mix stock or broth with porridge and lightly season with your favorite spices. Stir-fry a couple of veggies, or add some pickled veggies to accompany the meal. You can eat to total satisfaction; yet take in minimal calories and still get the nutrients you need including minerals. I think it is excellent for a crash diet. You

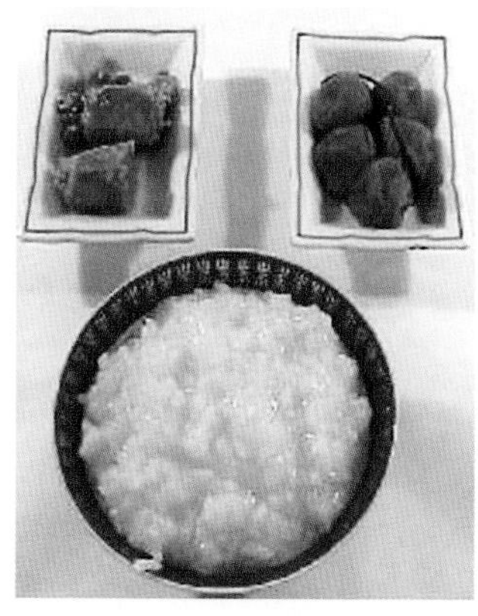

Soupy rice with umeboshi and preserved bean curd with a simple stir-fry veggie dish is ideal for a crash diet.

will be healthier and feel better during and after the diet.

Add stir-fried veggies and let them simmer with the broth and porridge as above. The porridge will have a nice vegetable flavor. As a matter of fact, cabbage porridge is one of the most common Taiwanese dishes. String beans, carrots, daikon radish, and most all vegetables taste good cooked this way. You can cut your veggies thin, shred them, or chunk them depending on the cooking time. Take it easy with the seasonings, especially salt. Even though we are eating a limited amount of food, we feel like we are eating a lot because porridge is mostly water.

Fancy Porridge

As you are cooking porridge, you can add other ingredients at different stages of cooking. For example, spare ribs or chicken with bones can be added in the beginning. The long-cooked bones will add more minerals, and the meat will break up giving the whole pot of porridge a 'meaty' flavor, which makes you feel satisfied, as if you had just eaten a meal of meat.

You can also add leftover meat. Shrimp or fresh fish taste great, and sweet corn or a can of Mexi-corn added to the cooking porridge gives it a sweet flavor and nice texture.

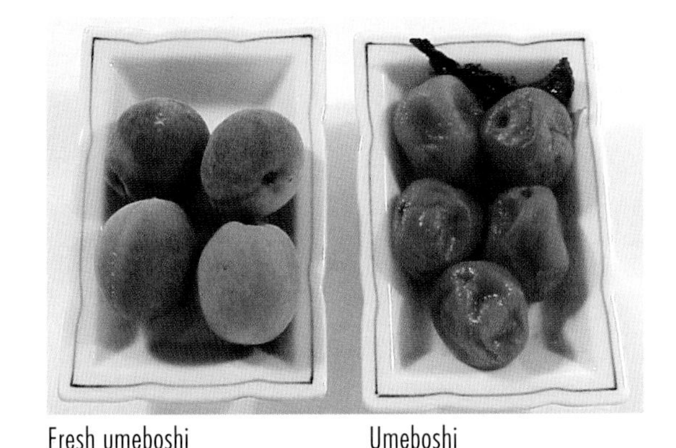

Fresh umeboshi Umeboshi

Light and Bland Porridge Meal

You've heard the term, "It makes my mouth water," right? When our body reacts to something mouth-watering, we secrete saliva, which signals us to eat and says the body is ready to digest the food. In a light and bland porridge meal, the porridge is best when unseasoned; just plain, simple, soupy cereal. How do we get the mouth-watering, then?

We accompany the plain porridge by very spicy, salty, and sour dishes, which taste good, but we don't eat in quantity. As an example, the Japanese have a pickled, sour plum called *umeboshi*, which comes in different flavors and tastes very sour and salty. The Taiwanese have preserved bean curd of different flavors for the same reason—and they're also very salty. We can enhance soupy rice, which tastes very mild, with a few dishes of stir-fried veggies. If we were to eat a couple spoonfuls of rice and then some veggies, we would respond to this food as tasting plain. To signal the body that we're getting something mouth-watering, eat something salty. We can pick up a very small amount of preserved bean curd or umeboshi to help spice up the food and encourage your appetite.

Ethnic groups all over the world, where the food is scarce and variety is lacking, have used this approach for eons. For example, some regions in Mexico and Szechwan province in China use very hot peppers in food preparation to compensate for the boring staple diet. In reality, we're actually eating a very small amount of salty, spicy foods in a light-and-bland meal. Preserved bean curd is about one-inch-by-one-inch, and we had no more than one to two per meal per person; and umeboshi is no bigger than a small plum or the size of a cherry tomato.

The whole idea is to create a bland taste inside the mouth and then stimulate the taste buds with very tasty foods that create chemicals in the saliva to help digestion. In the process, we enjoy a hearty meal with minimum salt intake. If you've never experienced this combination of foods, I assure you that it really tastes great. It's a very healthy way to help overcome a lifetime of overeating.

It may seem that making porridge and soup takes a good deal of time, and often it does, but you don't have to spend the whole time in the kitchen attending to the porridge. It is better to cook in large quantities, then divide into meal-sized portions, and store in the freezer for later. Package the porridge and soups carefully, so you can warm them easily in the microwave or steamer. You can take porridge to lunch at the office; just bring some pickles with it.

Dishes to Accompany Porridge

You can choose from a variety of dishes to serve with porridge including your own marinated or pickled veggies. There are plenty of items available in Asian markets. Try some of the following suggestions.

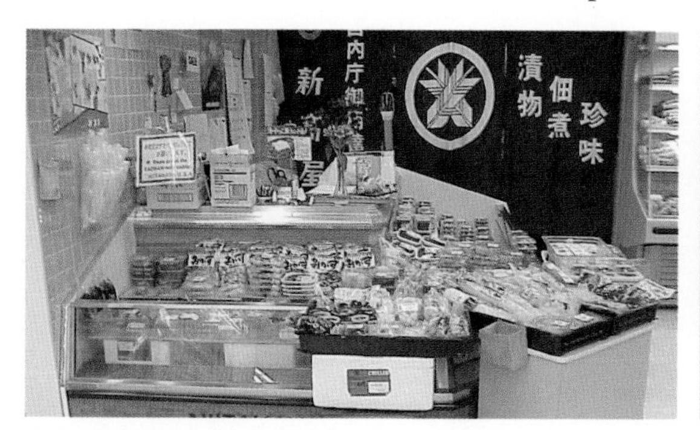

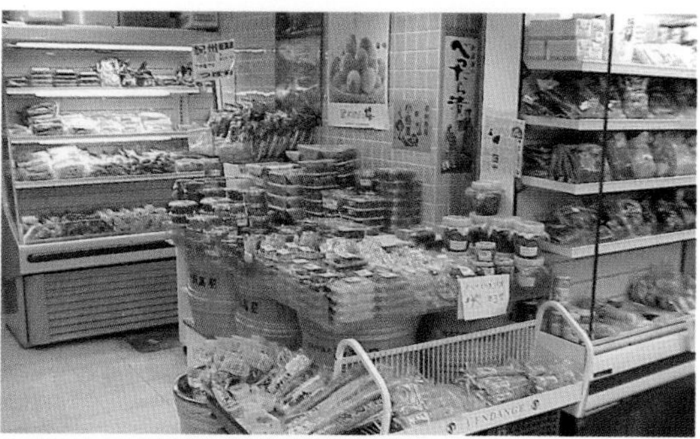

The photos above show a typical tsukemono (marinated and pickled vegetables) section in a Japanese market.

Canned Foods. Canned sardines or salmon are good with soupy rice. If you use canned fish, you don't need a meat dish. The fish should be served in small quantities. Did you know that fish contains omega-3 fatty acids, which promote cardiovascular health? According to the American Dietetic Association, for every 100 grams of raw fish, sardines contain 21.1 grams, Atlantic mackerel contains 2.5 grams, and salmon contains 1.2 grams of the omega-3 fatty acids. The bones taste great and also supply valuable minerals. Canned sardines taste delicious and come with all kinds of flavored sauces.

In addition, for ready-to-eat canned or bottled garnishes, there are many types of marinated or pickled vegetables in Asian markets. Some examples are shown in the photo below.

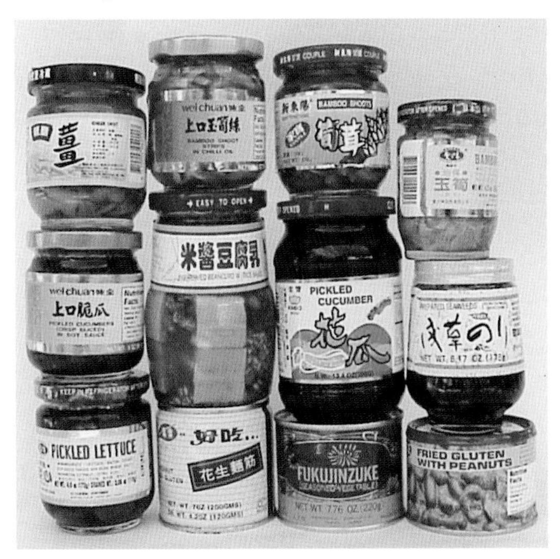

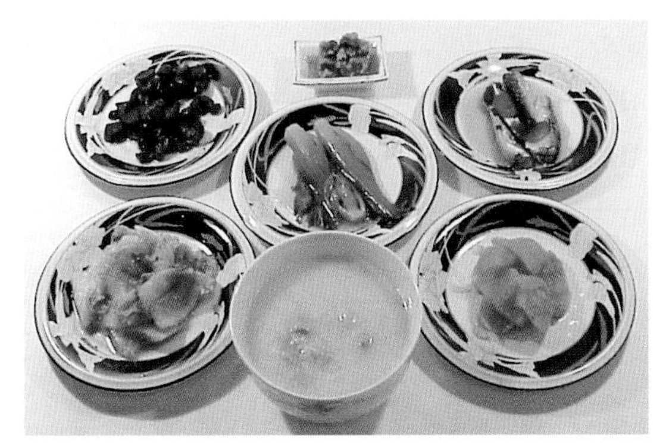

A delicious, fancy, and healthy meal. Clockwise from top left: pickled cucumbers, preserved bean curd, mustard, sardines, pickled daikon radishes (Takuan), chicken rice porridge, and kim chi.

Side Dishes. You can stir-fry one or two simple vegetable dishes to use as side dishes with your porridge and soups. Good dishes to accompany soupy rice are Japanese eggplant, onions sautéed with soy sauce, green onions stir-fried with chicken, pan-fried small fish, or a simple vegetable-tofu dish.

During the meal, eat the rice plain. Some people like to add soy sauce, but it is best to eat it plain. For every few bites of soupy rice, take a bite of one of the other foods. The plain taste of the rice makes pickled, salty food taste great, which stimulates the saliva flow.

As I mentioned before, if you're looking for a crash diet to lose a few pounds, this soupy rice diet is an excellent solution because you get the satisfaction of eating as much as you like. If you don't add cooked dishes, but just have pickled foods with the soupy rice, you'll have no oil and few calories. The soupy rice contains so much water, that you end up with very few calories.

Of course you won't eat 'light and bland' for every meal, but it's nice to do it once in a while. If we get that feeling that we'd like something to eat, but most food sounds too heavy; light and bland may be the answer. And as I've mentioned, it's a painless route to weight loss.

Although we Americans may not be accustomed to it, people from every culture have enjoyed this lighter approach to eating. I think you will enjoy it, too.

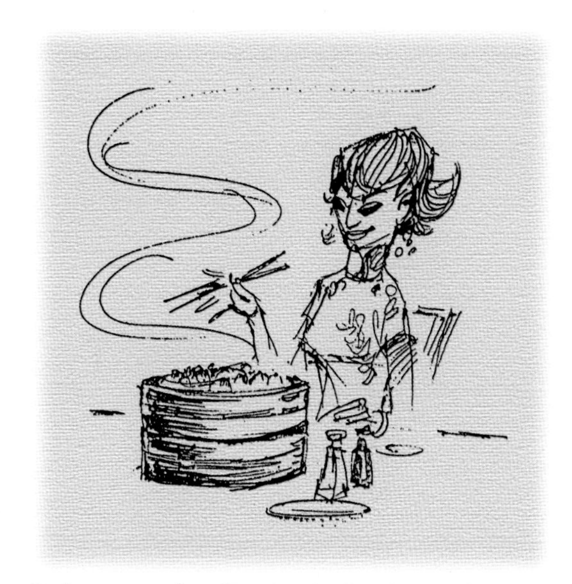

Little steamer dumpling. Succulent bits of meat in their natural juices are surrounded in a delicate envelope of dough and then steamed. This culinary item deserves worldwide acclaim.

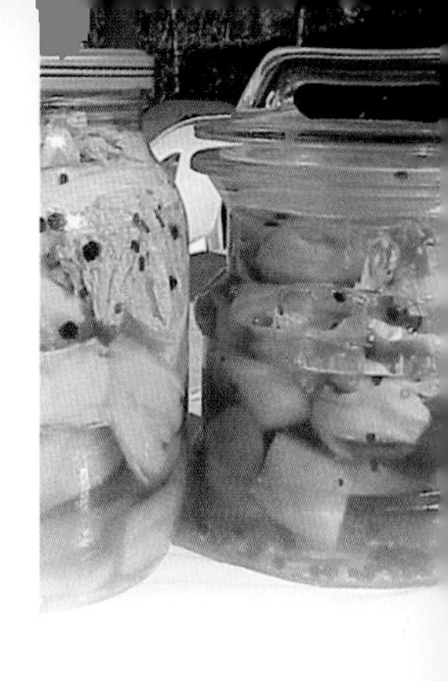

Chapter 12

Fermented and Marinated Vegetables

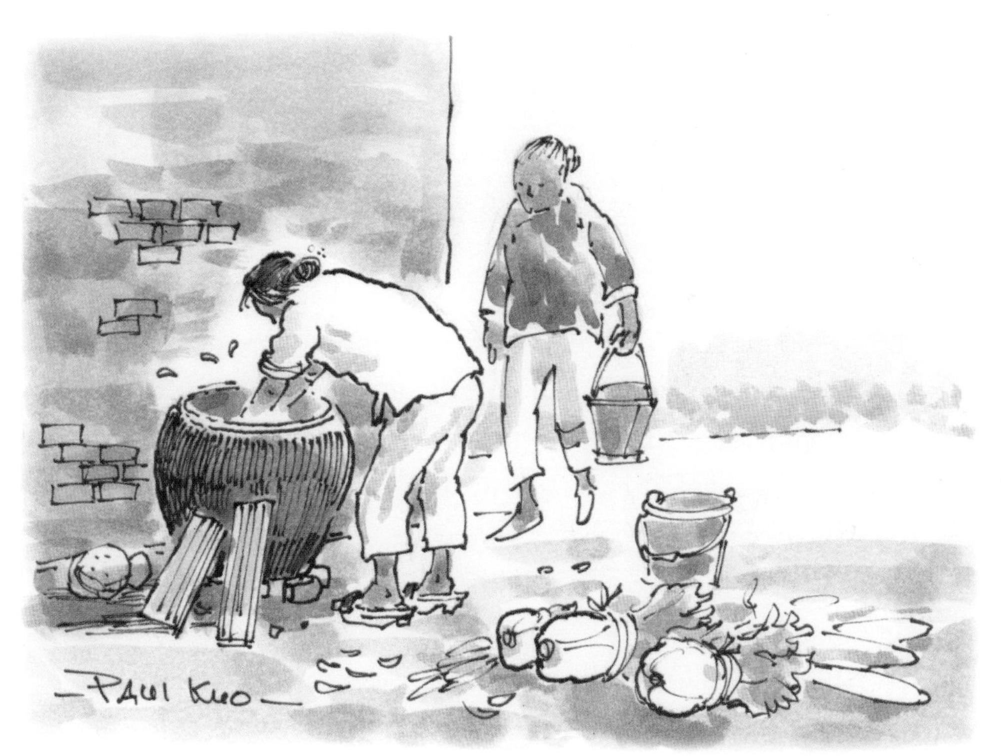

Traditional cultures around the world all feature some sort of fermented food. If you have dined in a Korean restaurant, you may have enjoyed *kim chee*; in Chinese cuisine, it is called *pau-tsai*, while the Japanese name is *tsukemono*.

In Europe, familiar fermented foods include sauerkraut, green tomatoes, cucumbers, beets, and turnips. A European meal would not be considered complete without a piece of cheese afterward.

Lacto-Fermentation: the Benefit of Lactobacilli

Most American supermarkets sell fast-processed pickles, which are made with salt, vinegar, artificial coloring, and preservatives. However, traditionally, pickles were always fermented. Before refrigeration and canning, most families preserved some of their vegetable harvest by fermentation; in addition to being a great way to preserve food, fermentation is proved to have many health benefits. The fermented vegetables are rich in lactobacilli, and their products improve digestion and increase our body's ability to absorb nutrients. Fermentation also produces enzymes, which are antibiotic, anticarcinogenic, helpful in digestion, and supportive to the immune system.

Medical researchers today point to green tea and soy products as the reason for the low cancer rate and longevity of the Japanese, but I think that the popularity of tsukemono is also an important factor. The Japanese consume more fermented foods than any other culture. In a typical Japanese market, you will always find a good section for Japanese pickles that are produced by fermentation.

The benefits of these stomach-friendly bugs are well recognized, and the National Institute of Health has been interested enough to fund scientists to conduct further studies on the subject. In the meantime, companies are pushing a range of foods and supplements packed with live microbes claiming that a daily dose of bugs helps preserve the balance of nature in your belly, aid digestion, and prevent illness. But some doubt these bugs can survive the hostile stomach acid environment to reach a useful destination in the intestines. So for now, it's wise to eat your homemade pickles.

How Does Fermentation Take Place?

Many species of bacteria are present on the surface of the roots of plants and their leaves growing near the ground. We know that the world is full of bacteria, some healthy and some dangerous. In fermentation, salt is used to inhibit the growth of putrefying bacteria, which allows healthy types of bacteria to propagate.

The lactobacilli on plants produce lacto-fermentation, which converts the starches and sugars in vegetables into lactic acid. This lactic acid is a natural preservative, which also inhibits the growth of putrefying bacteria (which can spoil the veggies) while allowing lactobacilli to continue to grow and ferment the vegetables.

As a Mouth-Watering Side Dish

Interestingly, in Taiwan, when you're coming down with a cold or under stress, traditional wisdom says to eat a 'light and bland' diet for a few days. This diet would eliminate meat, fats, and oils and, instead, have well-boiled soupy rice eaten with simple fermented vegetables such as Napa cabbage, regular cabbage, and cucumbers. This simple diet gives our body a break and allows the body's natural defense system to help bring our bodies back to health.

In a regular meal of rice porridge, pickled vegetables are served as side dishes.

They are not eaten in large quantities but rather as a condiment, flavored spicy, salty, hot, or sour. The first sight or even thought of these pickles makes the saliva flow, which improves digestion and helps us enjoy foods that may be light and bland.

You Have to Make Them to Get the Real Thing

Since you can buy pickles easily at the supermarket, why bother making them? As we mentioned above, most store pickles are quick-made with vinegar and salt and other additives resulting in a very acidic vinegar-tasting product without the health value of fermented food. If you've never had naturally fermented pickles, it may take a while to get used to the aroma and flavor of this natural food. For the most part, if we want fermented pickles, we need to make them ourselves or, hopefully, Grandma will send some for Christmas.

Basic Fermentation Principle

Pickling is very easy. Place your prepared vegetables in a container and add natural salt or salt water. Lacto-fermentation is an anaerobic process, which means that it takes place without oxygen and without being exposed to the air. But it seems to work fine in loosely covered containers. When you make homemade fermented pickles, be sure to leave a little space at the top of the container because fermentation produces carbon dioxide, which needs more space. Place your container at room temperature—ideally about 72 degrees Fahrenheit—for two to four days. During hot weather, it may take less time, while during cold weather, it may take longer to ferment. The pickles are ready to eat anytime after three days, but taste better when the fermentation has progressed sufficiently. You can store them in a cool, dark place—such as the top shelf of your fridge—for a long time. The flavor will get stronger over time. Some people like to mature sauerkraut for six months, for a mature flavor, but I think it's best to eat it as soon as it has the sauerkraut flavor.

The critical factor to pickling is salt. Generally speaking, use 6 teaspoons (30 cc or 2 tablespoon) of sea salt per 6 cups of water, or if you are on a low-sodium diet, use 2 teaspoons of salt and 2 teaspoons of whey, which contains lactobacilli (available at health food stores).

Veggies can lose their crunchiness and become soggy if too little salt is used. Use a glass jar with a tight cover, cover the veggies with salt water, and be sure to leave some space on top for expansion. Plastic or flexible jars don't work well because the slight pressure created by the fermentation can stretch the jar, and the cover can come loose.

You can add other ingredients beyond veggies based on the recipe; for example, traditional sauerkraut may also contain juniper berries, cumin seeds, and mustard seeds. Asian pickles typically include peppercorns, ginger root, hot red chilies, sugar, and so on. These additions are safe, but don't add meat, soy products, or other protein-containing ingredients. Protein additions require a special formulation.

The common vegetables used in Asian pickles are Napa cabbages, cabbages, carrots, and daikon radish. Pickling vegetables is as easy as stir-frying and just as flexible. Everyone seems to have a favorite combination and method. Just be sure that your vegetables, containers, and water are clean. I recommend using purified water for best results, but tap water will generally work.

Here's a typical recipe for fermented veggies:

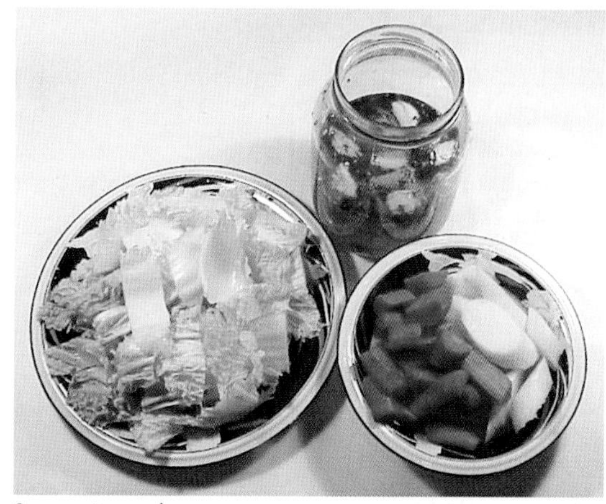

Get veggies ready

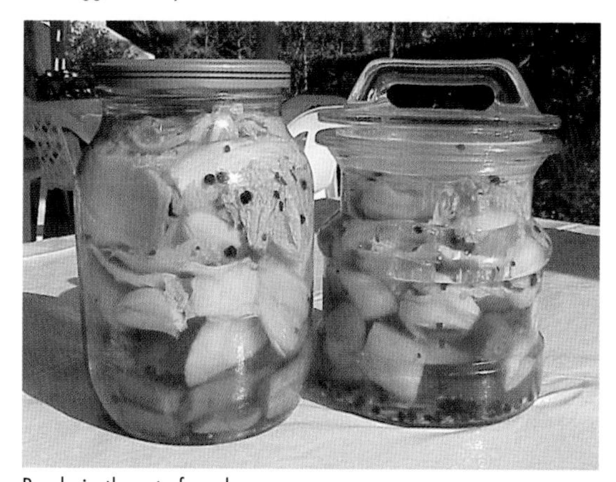

Ready in three-to-four days

Taiwanese Fermented Cabbage

1. Use 1/2-gallon (about 2 liters) glass or crockery container.
2. Seasonings, to taste:
   1 to 2 tablespoons peppercorns
   1 to 2 pieces crushed ginger (about 2 to 3 inches long)
   1 red chili pepper, whole or flaked, or jalapeño (optional).
3. Make a solution of 2 tablespoons of salt in 6 cups of water.
4. Add 1 to 5 tablespoons sugar (use at least one; more than 5 is okay if you like a sweet taste)
5. Add 2 to 3 large crushed garlic buds
6. And then add 1 to 2 tablespoons of white wine

(Note: One teaspoon is 5 cc; 1 tablespoon is 15 cc.)

Vegetables to use:

1. Cabbage or Napa cabbage with tight leaves, cut into 2- to 3-inch pieces
2. Carrots, peeled and cut 1/2 to 1 inch thick
3. Daikon radishes (white, long radish) peeled and cut 1/2 to 1 inch thick.

Cutting veggies this size preserves the crispness and crunchiness of the vegetables. Portions for each vegetable are at your discretion; generally, I use half Napa Cabbages, one-quarter daikon radishes, and one-quarter carrots for a good combination.

Preparation:

Put the carrots in the container first, then add the daikon, other ingredients, and then the cabbage; add one to two tablespoons of white wine. Top off with enough of the salt water you have prepared to cover the vegetables making sure you leave more than one inch of air space on top of the jar. Close with the lid and shake. Let it sit for four to six days at room temperature (four days in warm weather, six in cold). The water may become cloudy, which is an indication of the bacterial activity. By then, the cabbage should have a good flavor. You may notice that the daikon has a fizzy or effervescent quality, which many people prize.

As you can see, you'll learn by trial and error how to make this just the way you like it. Weigh and measure the ingredients and write your recipe down. The next time you can adjust the ingredients to suit your taste. Old pros used to make these pickles in big wooden tubs, covered with a cloth, and weighted on top. After fermentation was complete, they would transfer the pickles to smaller jars, tightly cover them, and place in cold storage.

It takes a little time to get accustomed to making pickles and using them in everyday meals. Once you get in the habit, though, you will find that they add immeasurably to the pleasure of your diet and, even more importantly, to your good health.

Marinated Vegetables

This is a dish you must try. It is simple, easy, and absolutely tastes great. You will never eat cucumbers and carrots with dip again. Marinated vegetables do not provide the nutritional advantages of fermentation, but they taste fresh and do not have the characteristic odor and acidity

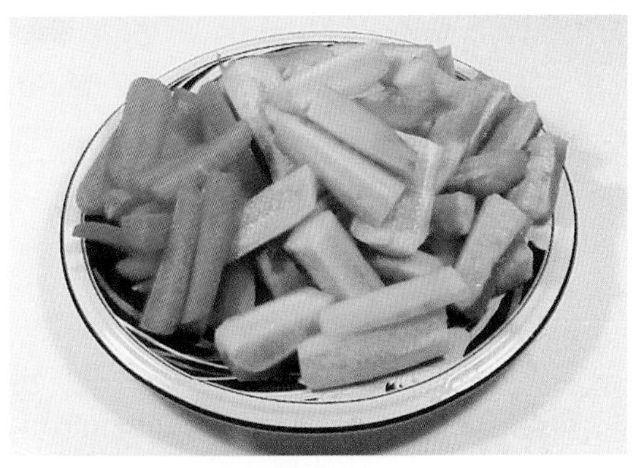

Cut carrots and pickling cucumbers

of fermented veggies. This is very popular with many Asian cultures where they use pickling cucumbers, daikon, carrots, hearts of broccoli, and many other vegetables including leafy vegetables.

There is no standard formula to marinate vegetables; people seem to have their own preferences. We'll show you here an example of a Taiwanese method of marinating pickling cucumbers. Pickling cucumbers are a little shorter and have more pronounced spines than the regular, large salad cucumbers commonly found in American salads.

Since they are often used for pickling, these cucumbers are not waxed, so they are not as shiny as the large salad cucumbers. Here's how to do it.

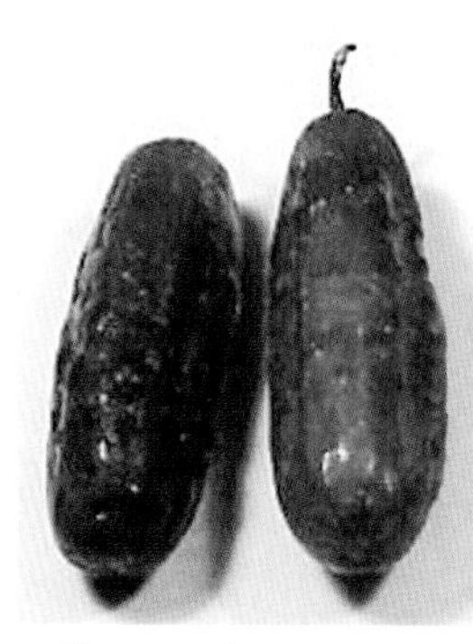

Pickling cucumbers

Simple and Delicious

1. Take 4 to 6 pickling cucumbers; prepare about 3 to 4 cups of cucumbers and carrots, approximately enough for a 5- to 6-cup bowl. Long, skinny cucumbers are better because they are less mature and have less seeds.
2. Remove the outer skin and cut off about 1/4-inch from both ends; if you omit this step, they can taste bitter.
3. Slice the cucumber lengthwise into four sections and then cut in the middle. You will have a cucumber sliced into eight pieces or more depending on the size.
4. Take another 6 pieces or more of peeled baby carrots, easy to find in your produce section. Quarter slice the carrots.
5. Place the cucumbers and carrots in a bowl; add 2 tablespoons of teriyaki sauce and 5 tablespoons of sugar (sugar will be dissolved into the juice and most is discarded later).
6. Add about one teaspoon of salt, 1 to 2 teaspoons of sesame oil, optional hot chili pepper flakes, 1 to 2 tablespoons of chopped garlic, and sweet rice vinegar. You can substitute ingredients to suit your preference; after a little experience, you'll know exactly what you like.
7. Put a cover on the jar and place it inside the fridge.

After ten to twenty-four hours, the veggies will be wilted but crisp, and covered with juice. The flavor is best when the veggies have marinated twenty-four hours. Taste after about eight hours and add salt or sugar to adjust the taste to your preference. Write down the ingredients and amounts for next time. You can keep these marinated veggies in the fridge for a week.

Broccoli Stems

Most of us cook and eat the flower part of broccoli and discard the stems. This is a shame because the stems are very nutritious, rich in fiber, and tasty, too. Just peel off the outer skin of the stem, then thin slice the heart of the peeled stem about one-eighth inch thick. Now the broccoli stems are ready to marinate.

Extra Dish for Every Meal

Marinated vegetables are normally served on a small dish at the beginning of a meal as an appetizer. These marinated veggies are better than raw cucumbers or salad because they're much easier to digest. The structure of the veggies is partially broken down by the marinating sauce.

Once you get used to marinating veggies, you will find it only takes about thirty minutes to make a big bowl. If you make it on the weekend, you can keep the marinated vegetables in the fridge to use during the week. They are very healthy, taste fresh, and are rich in fiber and nutrients. This is one form of veggies that your children may like! It's nice to know you always have one dish ready for any meal.

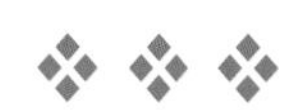

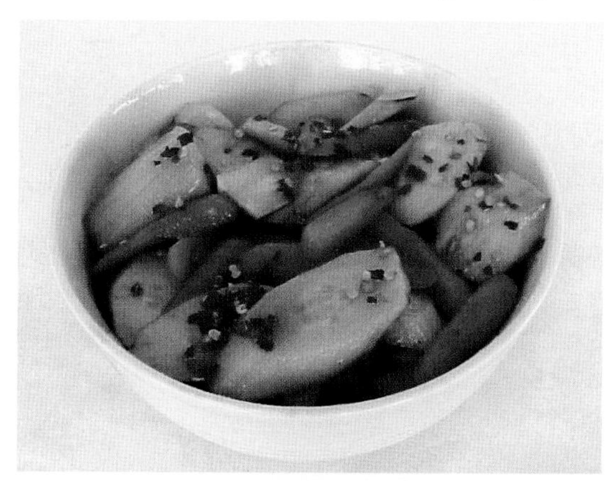

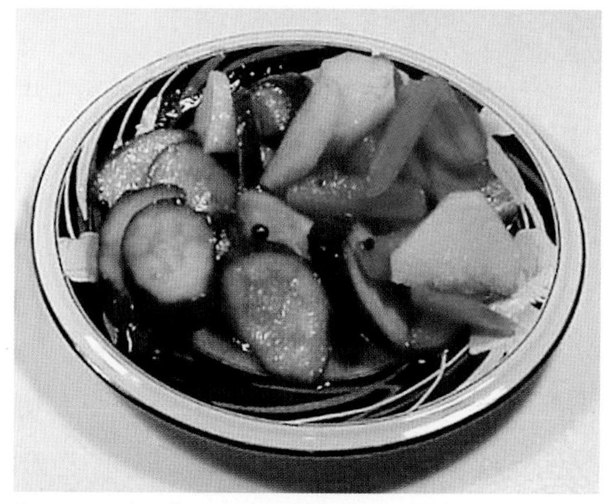

Some examples of marinated veggies

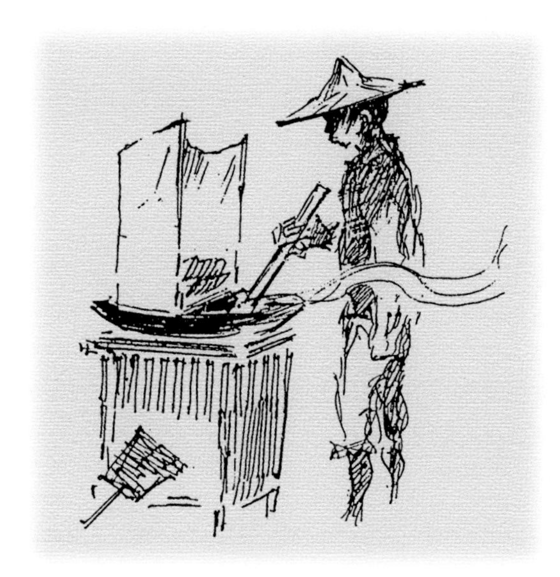

'Ch'ou Tou Fu.' Translated, the cry means stinking bean curd (preserved bean curd). It's sort of the limburger variety fried in deep fat and served with red hot pepper sauce. Formerly a great autumn favorite in Shanghai, it can be had all year round in Taiwan.

PART FIVE

Eating and Living in a Modern World

The advancement of science and technology in the twentieth century has transformed the average American's diet to something radically different from what our ancestors ate. Applying new technology and exercising the fundamental concepts of capitalism to produce foods cheaply and derive maximum profits, foods are now mass-produced, chemically processed, and widely distributed throughout the nation.

The increase in consumer demand for such foods by population growth and relentless, ubiquitous advertising to the young, coupled also with frequent family relocations and travel, has resulted in a sameness to the foods we seek and consume. Food items that are naturally grown and fall outside the pattern of brand names, restaurant chains, and commonly stocked grocery store shelves are becoming increasingly difficult to obtain, or have simply disappeared from the market.

Most Americans have become accustomed to relatively few, simple and sanitized, processed foods, eating such fares very selectively while totally afraid, or even resentful, of unfamiliar food. Let's consider an ugly incident in which the damaged US EP-3E reconnaissance plane was forced to land in an unfriendly airport on Hainan Island in China. When the ordeal was over, the crew members were interviewed by reporters about their treatment. They responded that everything was fine except the food was horrible: the Chinese served them chicken feet and fish heads!

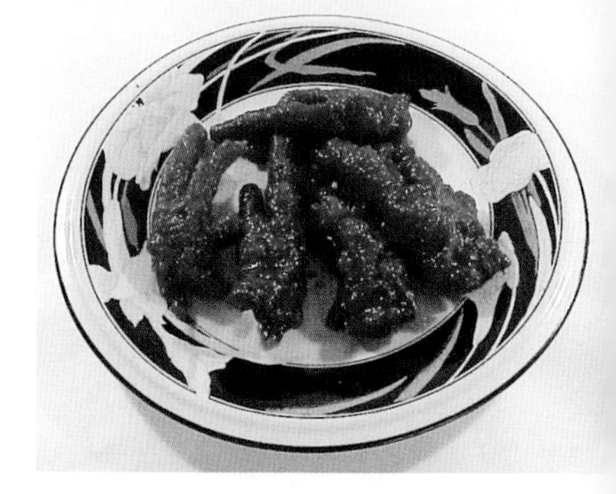

As I watched Tom Brokaw report that news, I realized it must have made Americans angry. We know (don't we?) that the communist Chinese are not as civilized as we are, but to feed unwelcome guests chicken feet and fish heads? How barbaric! But the fact is, the Chinese consider chicken feet and fish heads to be very tasty and wholesome dishes.

Chicken feet are held to be good for the joints. Chicken feet are also a normal and popular dish served in most respectable restaurants in Chinatown. As for the taste, it is indeed just a matter of taste. Captured Chinese crews might have exactly the same negative reaction to being fed Taco Bell bean burritos and a Pizza Supreme, though this would be heaven to a young American pilot.

As for fish heads, when our Taiwanese family had a fish dinner, the first thing we always did was to remove the fish head and place it on my mother's plate. I later joked with friends that the communist Chinese were not hospitable enough to serve our crew members a kind of fish stomach dish. If they had, they might have triggered World War III! There is a dried fish stomach that makes a good healthy soup, but costs about one hundred dollars a pound. In California, a bowl of soup with a few strips of fish stomach, cooked with chicken feet, mushrooms, and a few other choice ingredients cost about $30. No doubt, most Americans would prefer the Big Fish Sandwich Happy Meal for $5.

In America, an expensive dinner meal rarely exceeds $100 per person for the foods, excluding alcoholic beverages. In Asia, on the other hand, it is easy to spend over $1000 a person for the *food* only in an extravagant dinner for the wealthy. Asians have a penchant for rare and exotic food items that most Americans would not care for, and probably would not eat even on a dare or a bet! The point here is that the American diet has reached such a point of blandness and narrowness that even slight deviation and a hint of the exotic will turn up noses and turn over stomachs. Simply think back to the foods your grandmother or mother served you as a child, and compare that to what you can get a youngster to eat today.

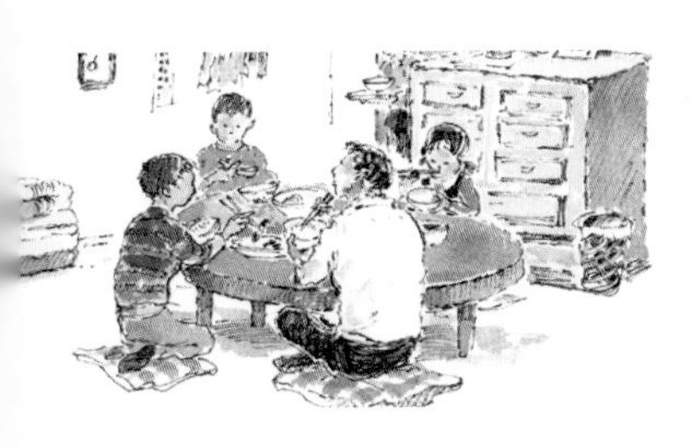

In **Chapter Thirteen** we take our newly acquired cooking techniques and put them into practical use. Eating is central to our existence and should be the most enjoyable aspect of living well. In our hectic modern life, we must admit, there is a minimal requirement to become better organized and carry out our plan of eating healthy instead of relying on fast and processed food. We will suggest some ideas for how to plan ahead weekly to accomplish this goal.

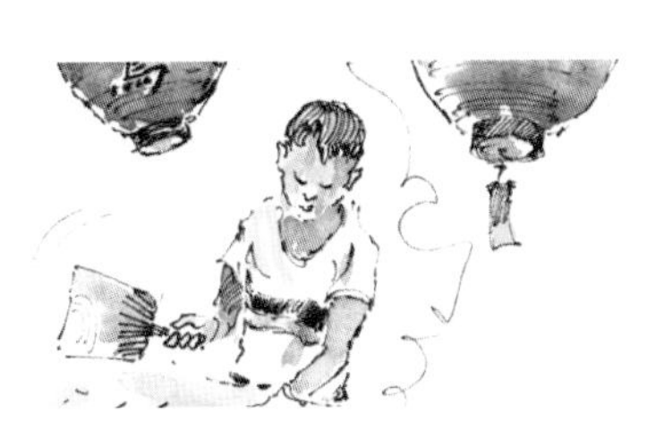

In **Chapter Fourteen** we discuss and introduce some good, wholesome food items not so familiar to most Americans, and encourage the readers of this book to be adventuresome and try new things. We re-emphasize the importance of eating a wide variety of food for our enhanced health.

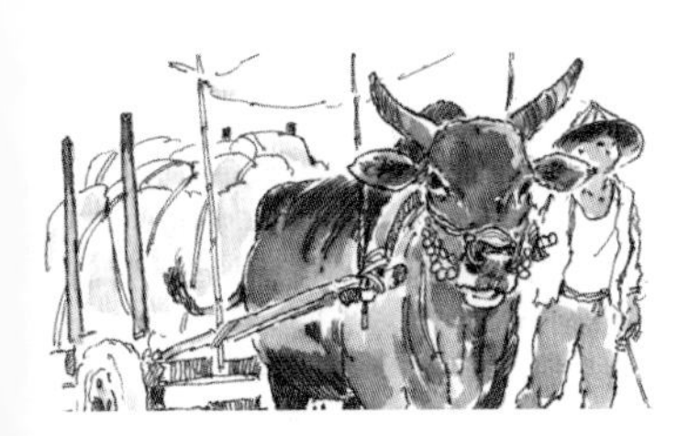

In **Chapter Fifteen** we take a look at the chemicals used in our homes. My professional career has involved dealing with hazardous chemicals. My book *Hazardous Gas Monitors* published by SciTech Publishing and McGraw-Hill is about detecting toxic and hazardous substances, and my professional concerns carry over to daily life. While we can achieve healthier lives through diet, the evidence suggests that we had better be mindful of our immediate environments and the dangerous chemicals that lurk there, as well.

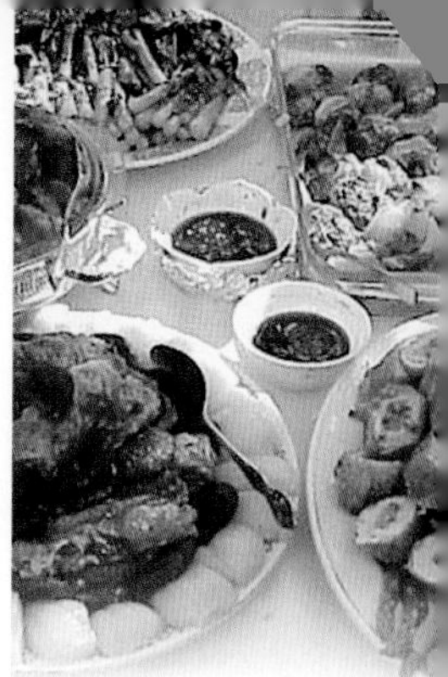

Chapter 13

Meal Time

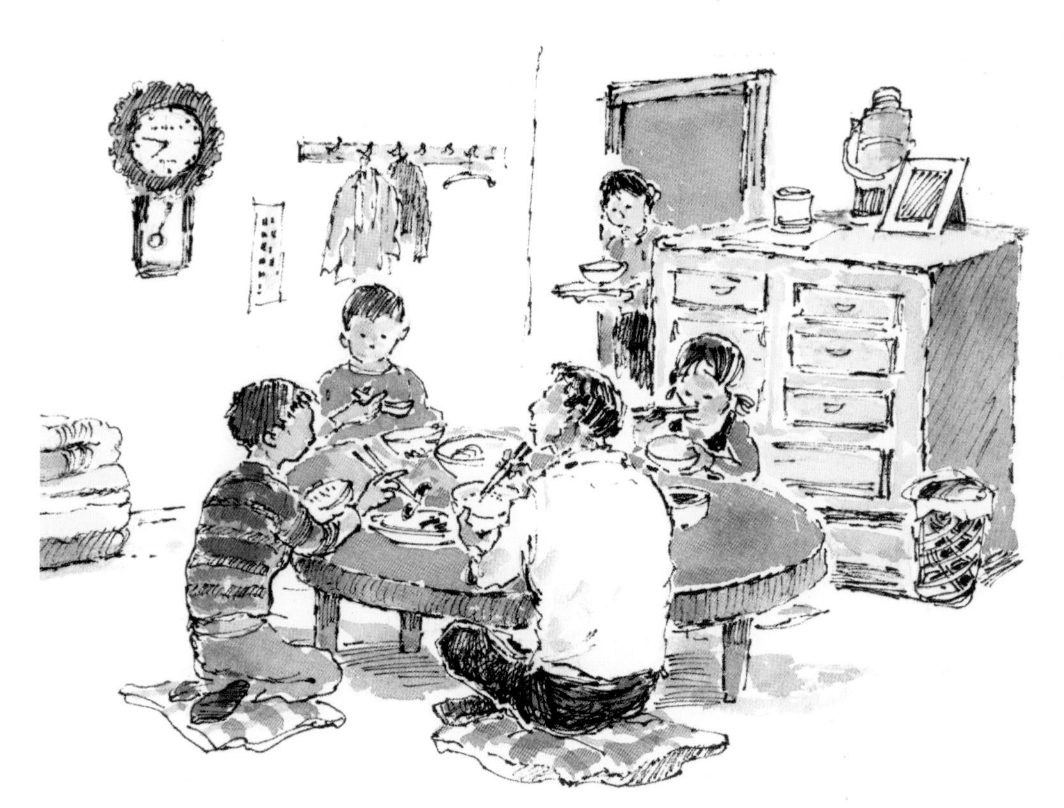

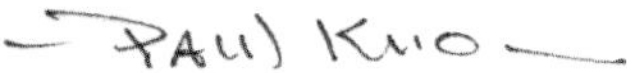

When it comes to changing the way we eat, most people would rather fight than switch. To an immigrant citizen like me, it seems amazing that America is such a big country, but people eat pretty much the same across the nation. You can sit down for Thanksgiving or Christmas dinner in California, Texas, or New York and get pretty much the same meal. In this affluent society, average Americans—rich or poor—eat just about the same foods.

If you ask people to change their diet, their response is usually something like this: "I've been eating the same way all my life; why should I change?" I can understand this—American food tastes okay and it's very convenient. It just may not be as wholesome and healthy, and most of us do need to make changes to improve our health.

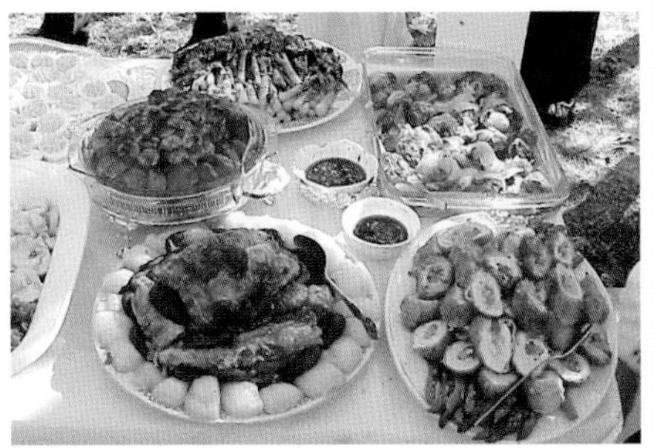
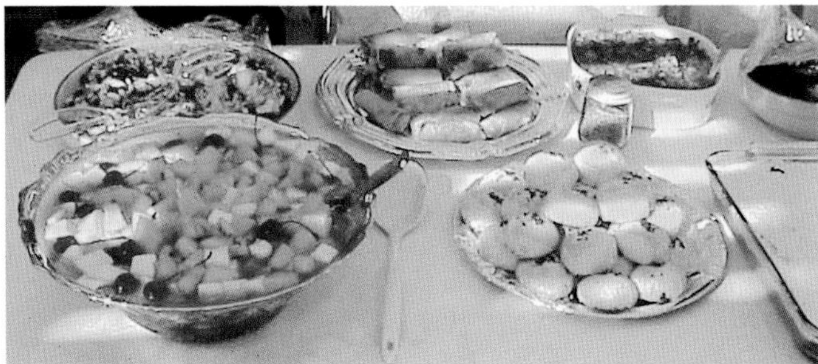

A typical Thanksgiving feast in my family includes turkey, cranberry and stuffing, and much more—twenty-five different dishes for forty people. Every year the dishes change, and we always expect the unexpected, but we always count on having turkey for Thanksgiving.

Differences in Food Choice

It's not easy to convince Americans to try new foods, let alone something strange or exotic. Very few of my American friends will even try seaweed or kelp, which Asians eat regularly and consider highly nutritious. Most Americans would choke if they tried to eat escargot, and most haven't tried caviar. On a recent trip to Charleston, S.C., during conversation, my host expressed great surprise that animal blood is edible.

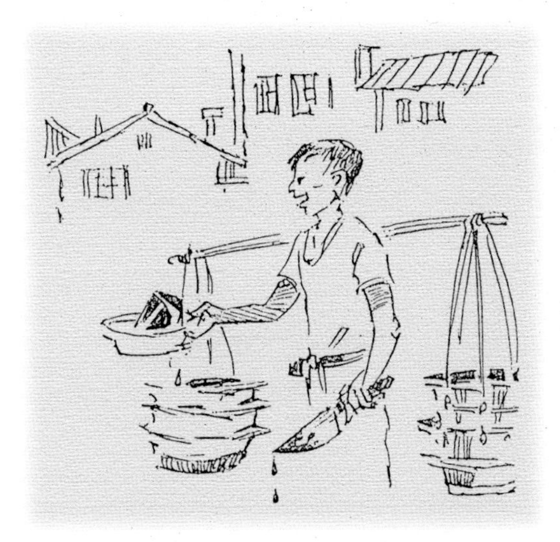

Blood pudding. Congealed pigs' blood is a delicacy around the world. In Taiwan, it is usually served with leeks as an appetizer.

He was in total disbelief when I told him his forefathers and relatives have, and still enjoy blood sausages, pudding, and other dishes cooked with animal blood and that his relatives in Europe still do.

I've noticed that typical Americans and Asians are a good combination living in the same community, as far as sharing what the market provides. In the meat market, for example, Asians believe, "The nearer the bone, the sweeter the meat." They believe dark meat is exercised muscle, and it tastes tender and sweet and also contains more nutrients. Dark meat is by far more popular among Asians.

In contrast, Americans are told white meat has less fat and, therefore, is better for you; most Americans favor white meat. Good combination, right? There's no problem in selling the whole chicken. The fact is that it's easy to produce chickens with a large breast, and since breast meat doesn't have bone, it's easier to cook; all around, white breast meat is easier to market. I doubt

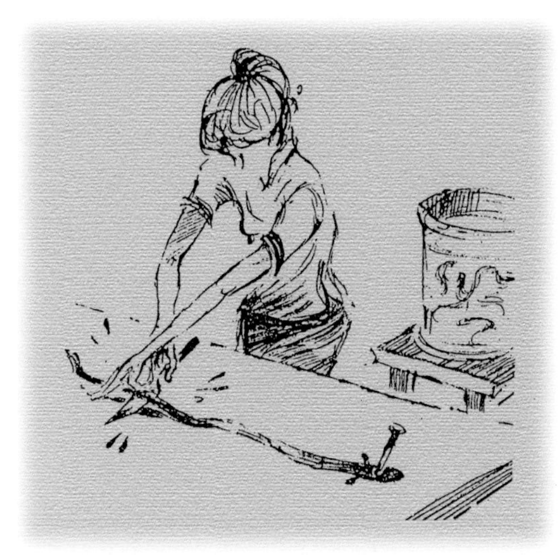

Filet of eel. Taiwan's famous food market offers a special treat of fried eels. One snicker-snack of a razor sharp knife and the deft maiden separates the meat from the backbone.

that the dark meat really has that much more fat, though, and most Asians eat smaller portions so the fat is not a problem.

Here is another example: Asians like small fish, and fish over about five pounds are not popular. You generally won't find salmon or halibut dishes in Chinese restaurants. In contrast, Americans like fish steaks from large fish, partly because they just don't want to deal with the bones. Asians love fish roe, which Americans throw away. Male crabs are larger than females; Americans buy male crabs while Asians buy females because they love the internal part of the female crab, which may contain eggs. From the ocean, sea urchins, sea cucumbers, jumbo clams, seaweed, kelp, and fish roe are good food—even delicacies—for Asians.

During a recent trip to Melbourne, Australia, I tried a type of local crab. A Chinese would call it King Crab. It was swimming in the restaurant aquarium, very big and dark red in color, and weighed about thirty to fifty pounds. I have only seen this type of crab in restaurants in Chinatown.

These foods would be unfamiliar to most Americans; however, things may be slowly changing. In recent years, I have noticed more and more people opening their minds to the pleasures of eating new things with much curiosity about international foods.

Now, I'm not saying that everybody needs to start eating strange, exotic food. Still, it's fun to learn something about these foods, and I recommend giving some of them a try if you get a chance. Mostly, I would say that it's a good idea to have some curiosity and willingness to try new things.

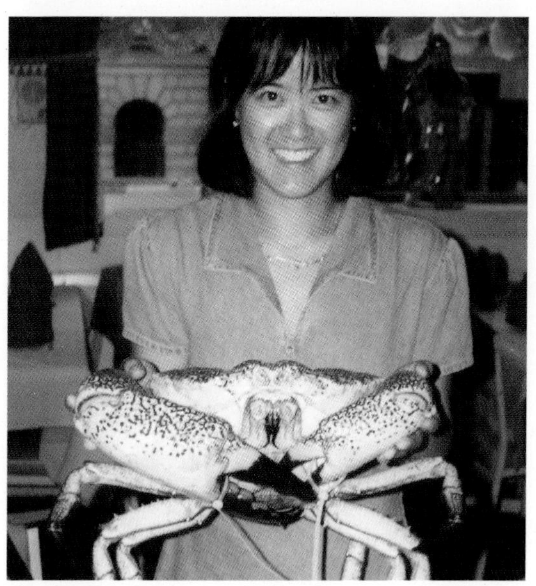

Tennis professional Kim Po serves up a King Crab.

An Endless Repertoire of Dishes

Hopefully, I have convinced you that eating a wide variety of food, as natural as possible, is the best way to achieve optimum health. You'll find the techniques illustrated so far are easy, even though different.

It is not unusual for a Chinese restaurant to offer more than a hundred different dishes on their menu. Some of the big restaurants in Chinatown offer 200 or more, plus their daily specials! In most cases, before you finish your first cup of tea, your order arrives. How is this possible? It's because Chinese cooks use a good basic technique, the one I'm giving you in this book. This flexibility allows Chinese restaurants to offer a rich selection of dishes prepared in record time. Of course, they prepare vegetables, meat, and all the other ingredients beforehand.

Perhaps we think that the cooks in such restaurants are well-trained professionals. Of course, there are many fine chefs in gourmet Chinese restaurants, especially in Chinatown, but for the most part, and for economic reasons, most restaurant cooks are ordinary people or the restaurant owners themselves. The average cook in a Chinese restaurant has minimal training—and is often not even Chinese!

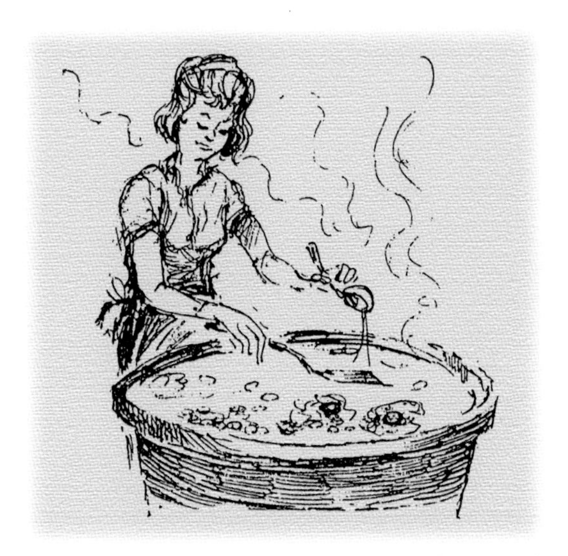

Fried oysters. Try this Taiwan delicacy at the famous 'Circle' north of the tracks. Midget oysters are fried on a hot griddle and basted with a mixture of egg and leeks. The resultant quasi-omelet is served with a native tomato sauce. This is one for the gourmands.

Knowing the basic cooking techniques should allow you to cook even better than a Chinese restaurant because restaurants are limited to purchasing only ingredients that are popular and profitable, while home cooks may have a much wider variety and can cook things to suit their particular taste.

To show you what I mean, in a popular, local Chinese restaurant, you can enjoy perhaps twenty chicken dishes including chicken with broccoli, chicken with dry red pepper and peanuts (called Kung-Pao chicken), chicken with snow peas and mushrooms, chicken with shiitake mushrooms and bamboo shoots, cashew nut chicken, chicken with vegetables, curried chicken, and so on. In essence, all of these dishes are prepared in just about the same way with little variation in the ingredients. At home, you can use cauliflower, cucumbers, cabbage, Napa cabbage, carrots, celery, eggplants, and green beans, and turn these 20 dishes into 200 dishes! Replacing the chicken with beef, pork, lamb, or seafood gives you that many more possibilities. There's no way we can run out of possibilities for delicious, interesting meals.

How to Eat a Meal

A Good, Old Fashioned Dinner

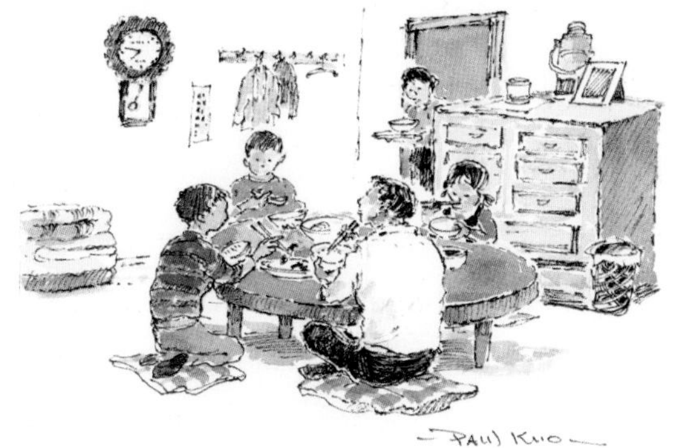

When I grew up, our family had eight children in the family, so there were ten people at our dining table. Taiwan was under Japanese occupation at that time, so our diets and lifestyles were a combination of Japanese and Taiwanese. We grew up without any modern conveniences: no refrigerator, no dishwasher, and no modern cooking range. We stored our leftovers in a wood cabinet with a copper wire screen. We didn't have running water in those early days, so every other day, the children helped fetch water from a nearby well; we stored the water in a large, pear-shaped clay container, which held about thirty or forty gallons. When we wanted water, we ladled it out with a large, hollowed-out dried squash sawed in half. My mother cooked on a stove made of clay, and lined with brick tile, in which we burned rice straw, rice hulls, sugarcane leaves, or any other combustible materials we could find. Occasionally, if we were fortunate, we enjoyed the luxury of burning wood.

There were two woks on the stove, a small one in the front and a large one in the back. In the large one, positioned directly next to the chimney, we boiled the drinking water, which was the only safe way to drink water.

My mother always started a meal by cooking rice, which took thirty minutes or more since the automatic rice cooker wasn't invented yet. When the rice was almost done, she'd stir-fry the vegetables. A typical dinner consisted of a soup, stewed meats, and three to four stir-fried veggies.

Our dinner table—about three feet by seven feet—was low like a coffee table, and we ate sitting on the floor, Japanese style. Men sat cross-legged and women sat with their knees bent, balanced on their shins (at that time, it was considered inappropriate for women to sit cross-legged). Many families had cotton-filled cushions to make this floor sitting custom more comfortable, but we couldn't afford that luxury.

The rice pot was placed next to my mother, who filled rice bowls for all of us. There was soup in the middle of the table, and three to five dishes of seasoned vegetables with meat along the side. Soup was a necessary dish because we didn't have juices, milk, or any other kind of drink to wash down the meal. Each member of the family had a pair of chopsticks and a bowl of rice. We ate by bringing the bowl close to our mouth and pushing the rice into our mouths with the chopsticks.

We also used our chopsticks to pick up food from the common dishes on the table. We'd eat a bite or two of rice, then a bite from the common dishes depending on how much food there was and how many people were eating. As a kid, I remember my mother would always eat slowly to make sure that the family got enough. Among us kids, we would signal each other and make sure there was enough left for our mother at the end of the meal. We filled up with rice; typically, a growing kid would eat three bowls of rice per meal making sure he got enough to carry him over to the next meal.

For most family meals, we usually enjoyed soups made of vegetables, meat and/or seafood. Miso soup, a kind of fermented soybean paste unique to the Japanese, was believed to be nutritious and aid digestion, and was frequently served. We always ate the soups hot. Sweetened or cold drinks were not considered healthy to eat with dinner; we'd usually drink them afterwards.

Interestingly, during a recent visit to Italy, I noticed that traditional restaurants had the same practice. We noticed Americans arguing with the waiters to get ice for their drinks. The waiters pointed out that ice melts and dilutes the beverage so it loses the original taste; besides, they said, ice is too cold, not good for you.

Modern Asian Meals

Today, Asian meals have changed a great deal. Each family member has a plate and chopsticks of his own. Each common dish comes with a serving spoon. Family members serve themselves with rice and the other dishes. There are usually plenty of leftovers, although sometimes, if there's a particularly delicious dish, it disappears rapidly. Half a bowl of rice is normal for most meals. At home, we usually prepare dishes with a few vegetables for a meal even for just two of us. Asians eat a wide variety of foods and, as I have said before, we believe that a wide variety of foods produces good health.

I also feel that eating together as a family in a leisurely way, enjoying each other's conversation, sharing food, and taking care of each other is a wonderful, civilized way to eat. By serving food from common dishes on a round table, it is easy to accommodate youngsters. It is normal, and expected, to see children in Chinese restaurants. If families ate together this way, I am sure that there would be less overweight, as well as happier, healthier family life.

Make Changes Gradually

No doubt, familiar foods are comforting like a security blanket. Drastically changing your daily diet can be difficult, and will probably fail. Instead, I'd recommend changing gradually. You can serve your normal familiar dishes, but add something new to complement the meal. You can also add some healthy ingredients—such as vegetables—to already-familiar dishes. A good example might be to add some carrots and celery to homemade chili, or to add stir-fried onions and small-cut zucchini to a favorite casserole. After a while, everybody will adjust to the changes. Don't be afraid to try new dishes; with a variety to choose from, I'm sure that your family will find things they like.

Plan a Week at a Time

Every meal should have some variety, of course. Some days you might have two to three dishes and some days, you might eat a little simpler with one to two dishes. Eat light and bland when you are under the weather or after just eating a series of rich and heavy meals. Serve marinated vegetables or fermented pickles with meals whenever possible. Drink anything natural with your meal, but no soda pop.

With this cooking method, you need to thin slice your meat for stir-fry. Over the weekend, slice meat to have it ready for weekdays. Divide the meat you buy into meal size portions and store in the freezer. This is an important first step. Thin slice the meat and marinate it with teriyaki sauce, chopped garlic, onions or green onions, olive oil, and wine, etc. Chemical reactions take place during the marinating process, which tenderizes the meat. It is better not to over season the food; it is much easier to adjust the taste at the end of cooking.

Divide the marinated meat into meal portions and save it in containers or baggies placed in the freezer. It is wise to date the bags, using them first in first out, and try to use them as fresh as possible. Marinate beef, chicken, veal, lamb, or shrimp; the more varieties, the more options you'll have when it's time to cook.

Prepare a large pot of soy sauce meat on the weekend; cook on low heat for an hour or so. Divide into serving portions and save in the freezer. For sandwich meat, don't cut the meat; large chunks of meat can be stewed and then sliced after cooking. On occasion, buy a package of corn beef brisket; follow the instructions on the package and add plenty of cabbage. This makes a great meal and the meat certainly makes good sandwiches. Try this once and you will never buy sandwich meat again.

As mentioned before, pre-cut and/or pre-mixed veggies from the produce department can save time. It is also wise to keep some frozen vegetables in the freezer. Everyday after dinner, think about what to eat tomorrow, and get ready for it. Fresh vegetables can be cleaned and peeled and made ready to cook for tomorrow. It is easier to cook dinner quickly, eat, and then do a little more work, if necessary. You can fix tomorrow's lunch at this same time.

A Weekly Planner

Here are some suggested weekly menus to illustrate what you could be having for dinner if you were to make a total change. However, in reality, you will probably want to make changes slowly by adding extra veggie dishes to your usual meals until you get accustomed to the changes.

Sunday

Stew a pot of meat (don't forget the daikon radishes and carrots) enough for two to three meals; divide it into serving containers, and save in the freezer. Marinate some pickled cucumbers and carrots or make kim chi. Stir-fry a couple of fresh vegetables and serve together with the stewed meat dish and fresh cooked rice for dinner. Cook enough rice for two days, and save the leftover rice in the refrigerator.

Monday

In the morning, place a Cornish game hen with carrots or daikon radishes in the rice cooker to make soy sauce-stewed chicken as described in the previous section; set your rice cooker to turn on five hours before you plan to sit down and eat dinner. Just before dinner, stir-fry the broccoli, then get the leftover rice from the fridge, add a tablespoon of water, cover and warm in the microwave for a couple of minutes. Sauce from the chicken is great to season the rice. Marinated veggies from Sunday should taste good tonight.

Tuesday

Place rice and frozen stewed meat (cooked Sunday) in the steamer. Set timer to start one hour before dinner. For a side dish, stir-fry cauliflower with bacon and stir-fry green beans with garlic; cauliflower and green beans can be fresh or frozen, or just use cauliflower only, and use marinated veggies in place of the green beans.

Wednesday

Stir-fry pre-mixed, pre-cut frozen vegetables with sliced meat from the freezer. Make a dish with extra sauce and thicken it with cornstarch. Place hot, steaming rice on the plate and cover with stir-fried veggies. Add another simple stir-fried bok choy or spinach dish if you want an additional vegetable.

Thursday

Use a pre-mixed, curry package and follow the instructions on the package. To cook a meat-curry dish, add potatoes and carrots or other vegetables with the meat. Stir-fry another vegetable dish for dinner.

Friday

Stir-fry two to three eggs (use egg whites only if you like), season lightly, and remove onto a plate. Next, stir-fry chopped onions and season lightly with teriyaki sauce; add eggs from the plate and stir/mix a few times. This is a light dish that the Japanese like. Stir-fry Napa cabbage with shrimp as a second dish. It is better to cook shrimp and cabbage separately, then mix after cooking, as with the eggs and onions dish. Each ingredient looks and tastes better this way. Alternatively, try a dish of leeks and beef cooked separately as above. Leeks come from the same family as garlic and add a great taste without the garlic odor. Wash the leeks carefully by slicing them open and washing each individual leaf with your finger or a brush; leeks sometimes have dirt tucked in between the leaves.

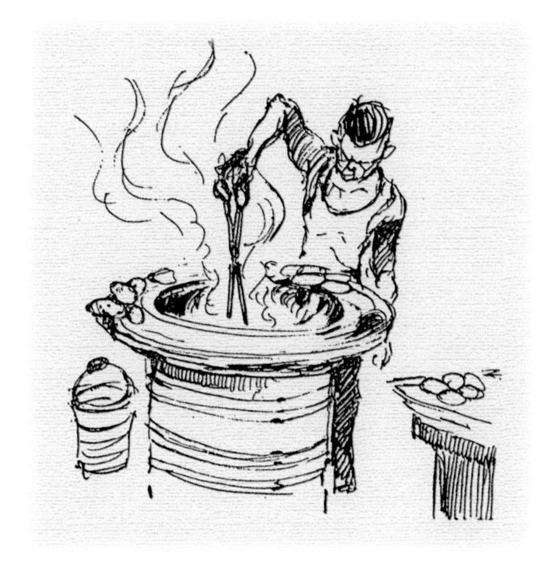

Ash can cookery. Shao Ping, Chinese hearth cakes, and soybean milk make a delicious breakfast. This street side specialty is made up of layers of flaky pastry and costs only five cents.

This is just a sample menu to help you get started creating your own dishes. I know that nobody can drastically change their eating habits, especially when you're feeding a family, so slowly and gradually add some new dishes into your daily meals and see how everyone reacts.

As previously mentioned, even if you order fast-food for dinner, stir-fry some veggies to eat with it. That way you can ask your youngsters to try some new dish and finish a small portion before they eat the divided-up fast-food. Some American families just place a teaspoon or so of a new dish on a child's plate to be finished by the end of the meal. Many kids grow up willing to try new things this way.

Breakfast

In America today, we can generally classify typical breakfasts into two types. One is the traditional eggs, bacon, and fried potatoes; the other is milk, cereal, and toast. The convenience and simplicity of breakfast cereals and toast are almost irresistible; they're getting popular in many other countries, especially metropolitan areas.

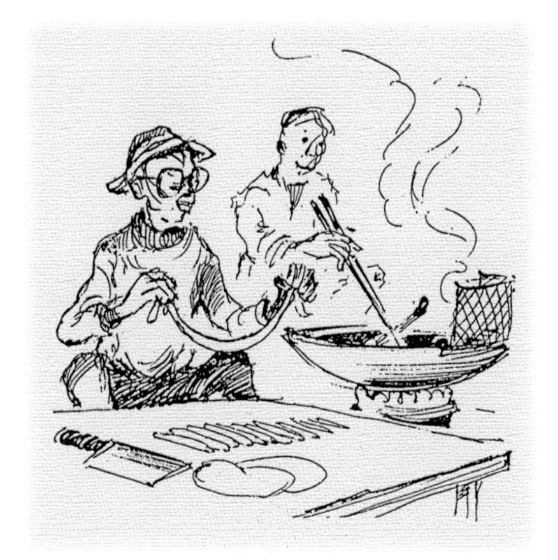

Coffee and........ 'Oil sticks' is the Chinglish equivalent for this tasty breakfast food. A cross between a cruller and a fritter, this critter is made of unsweetened dough and fried to crispy brown in deep fat. Try a pair with a hot bowl of soybean milk. "Twere paradise now."

Old wisdom taught us that we should eat something warm and light for breakfast. The food should be neutral, neither too yin nor too yang. For instance, in the old days, if I were going to drink orange juice for breakfast, my mother would have said orange juice is too sour and too yin for early in the morning. Bacon and sausage are too greasy. We should 'breakfast' gently.

A typical Taiwanese breakfast is plain soupy rice with two to three kinds of pickles. Eggs scrambled with onions are also a popular accompanying dish. On the street corner, you can always find fresh soybean milk and fresh plain pastries. The soybean milk is sweetened or seasoned mildly salty and accompanied with plain pastries. Today, toast and milk or soymilk is popular. There are many different kinds of hot cereals made of grains including toasted soybean powder, toasted rice bran, and wheat, etc.

To make drastic changes in breakfast are not easy. We might as well wisely eat what is available from the store. Some examples would include Shredded Wheat, Cheerios, Raisin Bran (and other bran cereals), and many choices from the 'natural' cold cereals on the grocery store shelf. Most people eat the same cereals all the time. It

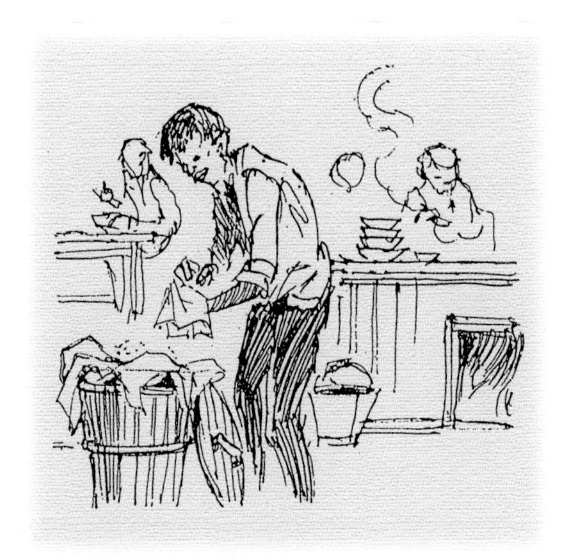

Quick lunch. This is the commuter's lunch. A big scoop of sticky rice is wrapped around a center of shredded pork. When squeezed into a hand-sized ball, it is ready for eating.

is better to change and rotate different kinds, which results in eating a variety of nutrients. Personally, I like breakfast with hot cereal and a little fruit. I find orange juice can be a little too sharp and my stomach is sensitive to it. On the other hand, papaya and melon are mild and comforting after the meal.

Lunch

In Taiwan, we never had hamburgers and hot dogs, and there wasn't any processed food available. Everyone carried a box lunch or 'ban-dong' to work, or to school, in place of our brown bag today. A ban-dong is a metal box, about four-by-six inches and a couple of inches high with a cover. Typically, it contained rice with a piece of meat and soy sauce; stewed, hard-boiled eggs; and some pickles. We ate the box lunch and then ran down the hallway to get a drink of the boiled water that the school provided. We had no concept of eating meals with a soda pop or ice cream in those days.

Today, to have a healthy lunch is a much easier task. Most workplaces provide a microwave oven and hot water, so it's easy to bring in a container of rice and another container of stir-fried veggies. It takes only a minute to warm up your food and make a cup of hot tea or coffee. Finish the meal with a piece of fruit. If you want to have a sandwich, it is easy to make and carry. Sandwiches can be improved by using stir-fried meat and veggies instead of

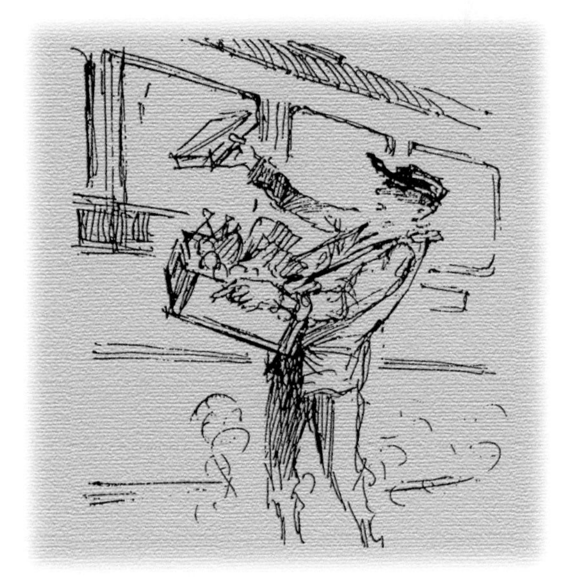

Trainside service. Nothing like the excitement of a train pulling into a station amid the cries of these platform vendors. Don't travel on an empty stomach. Duck eggs, oranges, and rice lunch boxes are only some of the nice things offered to the hungry traveler.

store-bought sandwich meat. When you plan meals during the weekend, be sure to remember to plan for lunches, too. Again, it's best not to have soda pop, chips, and candy for lunch.

We are so spoiled by the convenience of fast and processed foods, that most of us don't worry about what we are having for dinner until thirty minutes before it's time to eat. There are plenty of backups on every street corner in case we don't get dinner cooked. Like just about anything else, mealtime works best if we plan ahead. We need to include breakfast, lunch, and dinner in the plan. Fortunately, with the broad guidelines I have given you in this book, you can prepare a number of possible foods so there will be plenty of quickly-prepared choices for dinnertime.

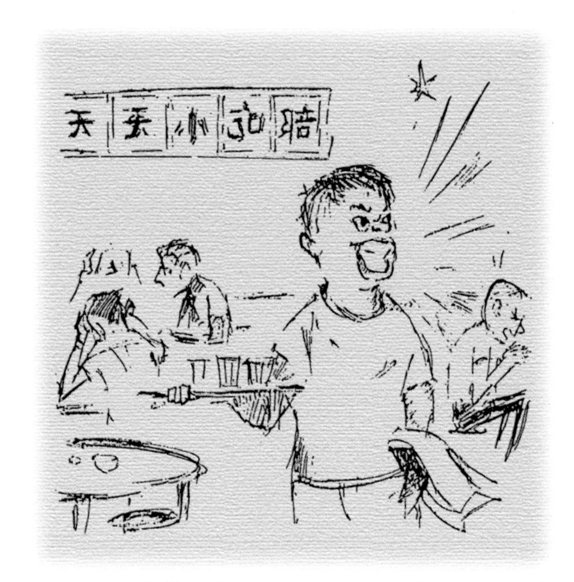

"One meat ball!" That last scream you heard was not a call for the cops or the fire engines. It was just the waiter at the corner lunchroom announcing your order to the cook. When you leave, he will call out the amount of your tip over the same intercom.

How to Eat Out and Stay Healthy

Most of us eat out regularly, often just for fun. Since eating out is such an important part of our modern life, it is important to follow a few rules so we can enjoy the food and still remain healthy.

Stay Away from Deep-Fried Food

Take a look at any coffee shop menu and you will see that about ninety percent or more of what's offered is deep-fried. Deep-fryers are standard equipment in many establishments, and they use a specially processed, commercial oil that doesn't change color when heated to higher temperatures. Deep-frying basically boils food in oil. The high temperature of the oil evaporates the water on the surface of the food and slightly burns it, which gives it that special smell and crispy texture.

Frying in oil disguises the taste of foods; for example, deep-fried fish doesn't taste fishy because of the frying process. Deep-frying adds many calories as well as unhealthy oil to the diet—and any oil becomes unhealthy when it's overheated or reheated. It's wise to minimize or eliminate deep-fried foods including french fries and onion rings.

Don't Drink Soda

As we have seen, soda pop is made from sugar and chemicals—all of which drain your good health. Drink plenty of water instead. I always ask for water with lemon, so I can squeeze the lemon into my water for a pleasant mealtime beverage. Recent studies show that your blood sugar rises more slowly—which helps with weight loss—when you have lemon or vinegar with your meal.

Start with the Veggies

Most restaurant vegetables don't taste very good so you need to eat them while you are still hungry. Ask for a side dish of vegetables and request that they not be overcooked. Don't be afraid to ask for a box; in fact, in most cases, if you don't take some food home, you probably ate too much.

Choose a Good Restaurant

A colorful menu full of deep-fried food is a good hint that you need to be careful. Take a good look at the patrons in a restaurant; if a high portion of them are overweight, and you don't want to look like them, you are probably in the wrong restaurant. Remember, restaurants are in business, which means the only measure of their well-being is how busy the cash register is. Restaurant menus are designed for good business, not your health or waistline. We need to exercise our good common sense and judgment.

Don't Assume Any Ethnic Restaurant is Healthier

By simply going to an ethnic restaurant, don't assume you're eating healthy; that can be a mistake. For instance, a Chinese restaurant in Chinatown is very different than a Chinese restaurant that caters to the general public. Restaurant owners always adjust their cooking to suit local tastes. They just want a successful business. Many ethnic restaurants have two sets of menus, one for the traditional population, and the other for non-ethnic customers.

There are basically two categories of cuisine, continental and island. Continental cuisines such as European and Chinese are rich and often complex and sophisticated. They serve hearty foods that can please many different tastes. Most restaurants in America are good examples of continental restaurants. Island cuisines, on the other hand, aim to appeal to their particular population. They are difficult to adapt to popular tastes. Take Japanese food, for example. Typically, this food is too exotic and the recipes are too cumbersome for American tastes. They use specific, unusual ingredients such as seaweed and rare vegetables. When we Americans eat Japanese food, we're having a few adapted dishes suited for American tastes.

So when you eat at a Japanese restaurant, most of the time you are enjoying dishes adapted to continental-style cooking. In the past in Japan, you would rarely eat meat from animals with four legs; that was considered somewhat barbaric. And traditional Oriental cookery never includes dairy products.

Some restaurant 'imports' have brought great food choices to America. For example, about the same time Toyota was introduced into America, chefs invented Teppan Yaki, which is similar to the Mongolian barbecue where a chef cooks a patron's chosen foods on a large, hot grill in front of the patron. Often the chef handles the cooking with a flourish to entertain the guests, and most of these dishes contain good amounts of veggies.

A similar presentation is the Korean barbecue, where marinated meat is cooked at the table with a butane stove; in California, it's called Korean barbecue, but in Korea, it's called California barbecue. As you are beginning to see, many popularized Oriental foods are actually adaptations for the American public. If you want to taste some real Oriental cooking, make friends with someone from the East and learn from them.

Order Simple Dishes (It's Healthier and Usually Cheaper, too)

Order food that's simple, plain, and wholesome with a cooking method that's quick and simple. This rule is important for those who dine out a lot. Of course, on occasion, you'll decide to go for broke and enjoy some of the richer pleasures of life, but most of the time, try simple.

Try a New Place

Most of us go to just a few restaurants regularly, but it can be a real adventure to branch out and try something new. It's our human nature to stay within familiar patterns—we like our comfort zones—but you might like to experiment and try some new tastes. Trying different foods also gives us a wider range of nutrients.

On many occasions, when we have Hindu visitors from India, we order dishes without meat in Chinese restaurants. Chinese chefs are accustomed to requests for vegetarian foods and will gladly prepare vegetarian dishes. Next time you go for Chinese food, tell them you are a vegetarian and request a vegetable soup and vegetarian dishes, no deep-fry, just light and bland. Generally, as a rule, one dish per

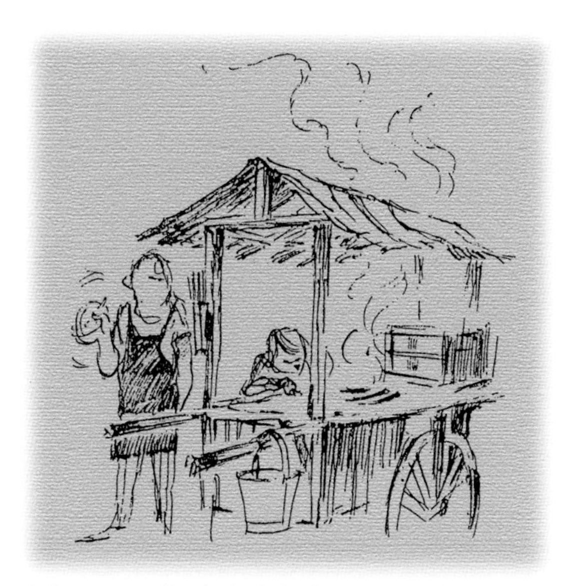

Nighttime snack. 'Clank, clank, clank!' The midnight sound of spoon on bowl signals the arrival of the man selling fish ball soup, a light treat guaranteed not to cause insomnia or nightmares.

person is plenty, or four to five dishes for six people. You will be surprised how hearty the meal can be. You will feel great after the meal and find that it's less expensive.

Conclusion and Checklists

You're probably convinced by now that it's good to eat a variety of natural, fresh, simple foods. Using this book, I hope you can create this kind of diet for yourself and your family, and enjoy good health and great food at the same time. True, you'll probably end up changing your lifestyle somewhat, but I anticipate that you'll find the changes easy and natural.

Remember that the body is a very complex biological system with a built-in clock. For example, it's healthy to get sleepy when it's time to go to bed. Eating works the same way; it's good to eat three meals at about the same time everyday. It is best not to surprise your body with unexpected meals. If you need something between meals, try not to shock your body with high-sugar snacks such as candy. Try fresh fruit instead, or perhaps a handful of nuts or seeds. A cup of nice hot tea can eliminate between-meal cravings and also help you feel satisfied. If you are trying to get over bad eating habits, you may be happy to learn that it only takes two to three days to overcome a habit and start anew.

Once you change your diet, make sure your energy and stamina have improved. Additionally, using a good bathroom scale, weigh yourself at the same time of the day everyday and write it down. As you monitor your weight, you'll probably see a slow, steady rate of loss; that's the healthiest way to lose weight. If you are eating healthy and your weight doesn't change in a few weeks, try eating less. Studies have consistently shown that taking in fewer calories is the best way to lose weight, and it keeps you healthy, too.

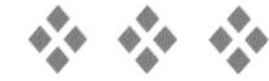

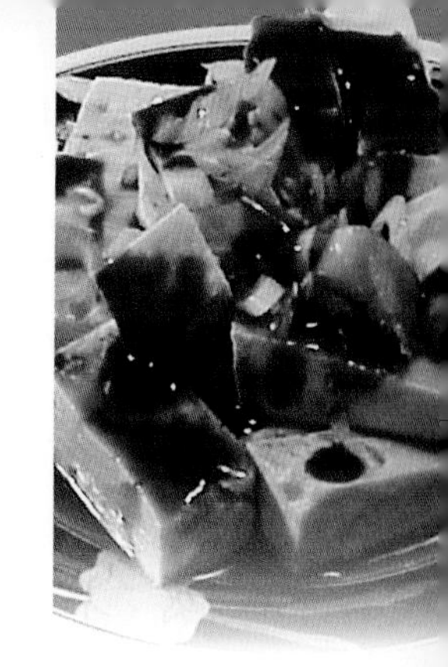

Chapter 14

Unfamiliar Foods

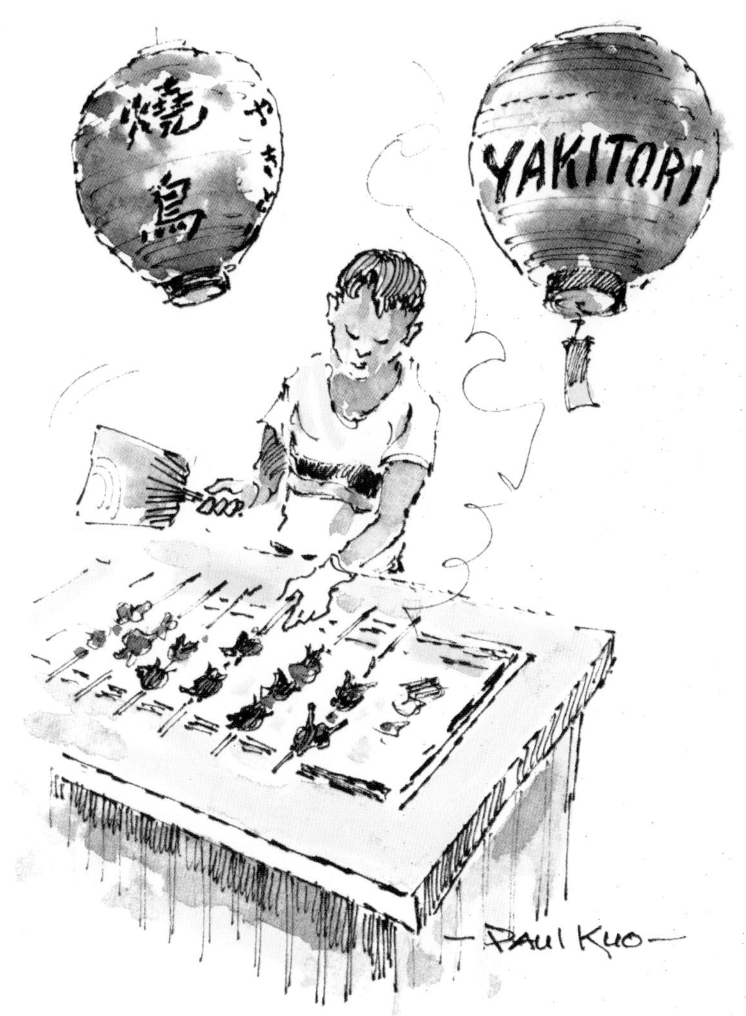

As we discussed in our chapter on 'shrimp mentality,' today most of us eat instant, refined, sanitized foods. In fact, most of us are just a little bit spoiled. We have grown up watching enough commercials to be conditioned to know what we *think* we like, and there's always somebody out there to sell it to us. Unfortunately, these processed foods don't supply our entire nutritional needs. Instead, they overload our systems with unwanted calories and chemicals, as well. We are missing elements from foods that are not marketable or that are difficult to process for the market. These types of foods are not pushed by processors with enormous advertising budgets, so we think we don't like them.

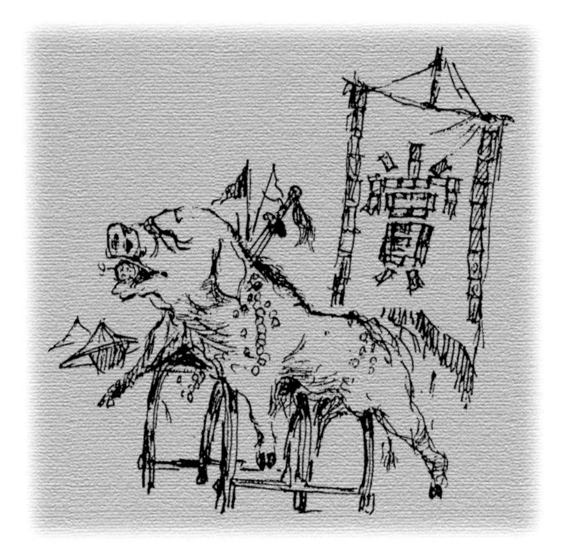

Pyrrhic victory. This porker made a pig of himself and ended up with the first prize, nicely outlined in ten-dollar bills on the banner. From his position on the high hurdle, he presides over the local 'pai pai' (religious ceremony) until he is cut up to feed the assembled guests.

Mother's Buddhist Philosophy

In the old days, our mothers used to say that if we were going to sacrifice a life for our food, we were obligated to eat the whole edible portion of the animal. She said it was unethical to throw edible parts away and if we did, we would be punished and struck by lighting. We have dishes for blood, intestines, and most of the organs.

When I tell this to my American friends, most shake their heads in disbelief that people could eat an animal's internal organs. The fact is that people from all over the world do it. Modern Americans are the only people who don't, as a rule, recycle these parts. And you probably know that this can be the problem with mad cow disease, because the unused parts are made into protein supplements for cattle feed, concentrating the mad cow pathogen.

I don't intend to become unpopular with my American friends by trying to convince them to eat animals' internal organs. If we look a little further, there are a number of more friendly foods that may seem unfamiliar but, after a little getting used to, can add important health-building elements to our diet.

Should We Eat Just Meat?

Endocrinologists at the University of San Francisco have found that the typical protein-rich American diet overloads our body with acid. Protein contains sulfur, which our livers turn into sulfuric acid. The body has to neutralize some of it by looting the bones. The body may have to resort to stripping calcium from our bones to help reduce the acidity in our systems causing hip fractures, osteoporosis, and related problems.

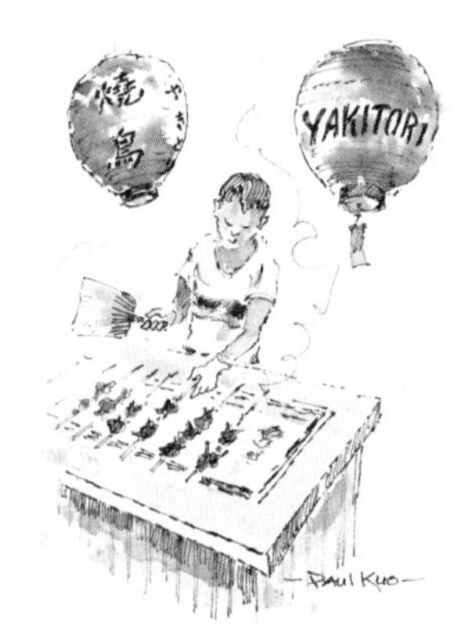

Eating meat with edible bones may solve this problem. As an example, a Japanese style snack called *yakitori* was popular in Taiwan.

Sparrows. There were plenty of sparrows in the rice fields, especially during the rice-harvesting season. Sparrows were caught, cleaned, and marinated in soy sauce and vinegar, and then grilled. Roasted sparrow is delicious and one eats the meat and bone together with sake or beer. This dish has the complete nutrients a bird has to offer. Today, chemical farming has decimated the sparrow population and yakitori has become very expensive when available. Instead, in the restaurants, yakitori has become grilled chicken breast.

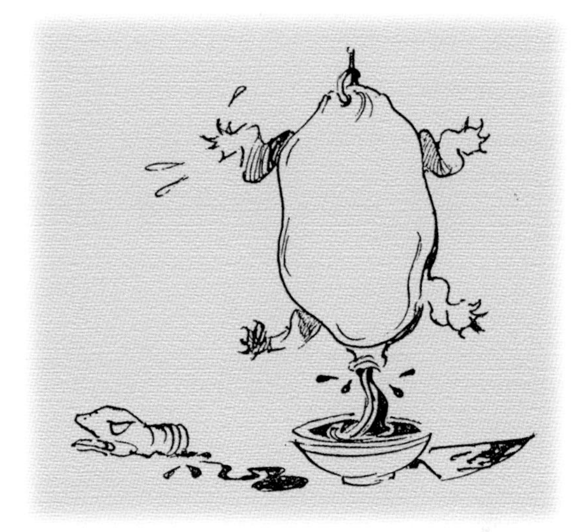

Step right up. The blood of a special soft-shell turtle, *Trionyx sinensis*, is very dear. In some medicine shops, a drink of this panacea costs NT $200. On top of that, the head of the ungraceful animal still bites after it's cut off.

Tiny Fish. There are also many kinds of tiny fish in Asian dishes. These small fish are eaten whole since the bones are soft and edible. As an example, capelin fish, which are about four-inches long and full of roe, is a popular side dish; the Japanese call it *shishamo*. If you go to a traditional Asian restaurant with an Oriental friend, have him order a dish of small fish for you. You will be delighted at how delicious they actually are.

The Power of Soy

When most Americans think of soy, they think of Japan. You might be surprised to learn that America is the biggest producer of soybeans in the world. In the

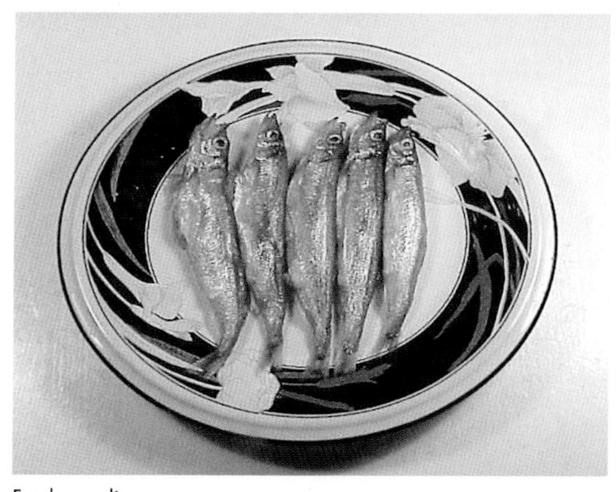

Fresh capelin

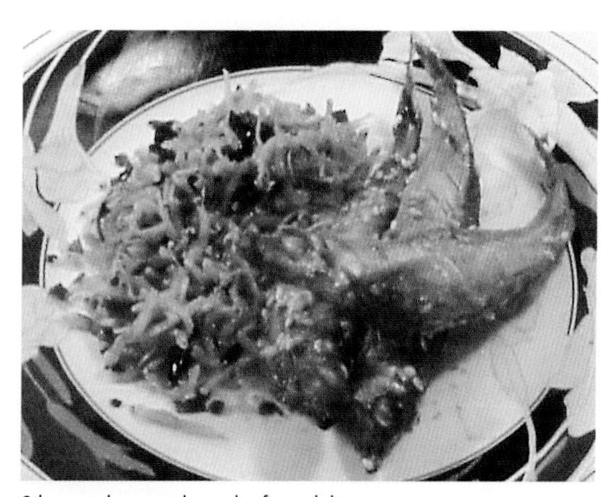

Silver anchovy and capelin from deli

Orient, soy products are a very important part of the diet and are an important source of protein, while in the West, farmers feed the soybeans to animals and then eat the animals.

I think that's a pity because soybeans are rich in vegetable protein and contain the most complete vegetable proteins of all the plant products. In the Orient, soy has been used as a main protein source—instead of meat and dairy products—for thousands of years.

Soy is the only commonly available vegetable food with all eight of the essential amino acids, which makes soybeans comparable to meat, dairy products, and eggs. They contain good fat, lots of fiber, and vitamins and minerals as well, and do not contain cholesterol. Soy protects our cardiovascular system by lowering the bad cholesterol and raising the good cholesterol. It protects the arteries from free radical damage, prevents plaque from sticking to arterial walls, and prevents blood clotting. As you can see, eating soy products may reduce the chance of heart attacks and strokes.

In addition, soybeans are rich in phytoestrogens. These plant compounds aren't estrogen, but they have estrogen-like properties and can balance a woman's estrogen either by augmenting or suppressing it. No drug can do this; it is the action of a natural compound in soybeans. When natural estrogen levels in the body are low, as during menopause, phytoestrogens mimic estrogen to relieve typical symptoms associated with menopause. When estrogen levels are high, phytoestrogens can reduce the excess estrogen. Eating soy products can naturally and gently balance the hormone levels in the body. Most Asian women who regularly eat soy products do not experience the menopausal symptoms such as hot flashes, moodiness, and excessive anxiety that others do.

Recently published studies show that soy keeps circulating levels of estrogen low, which in turn inhibits breast cells from becoming cancerous. Women who drank more than four glasses of soy milk a day, for one month, had their peak blood levels of estrogen drop 40 percent.

In addition, soybeans have powerful, cancer-fighting and cancer-preventive properties. These research findings are very exciting, and I anticipate that there will be many more discoveries about soy.

So how do you add soybeans to your diet? Over thousands of years, the Chinese have developed very sophisticated methods of preparing soybeans from soy sauce to tofu. Many still claim to have secret formulas and processes for the finest soy products. I feel that the basic way to consume

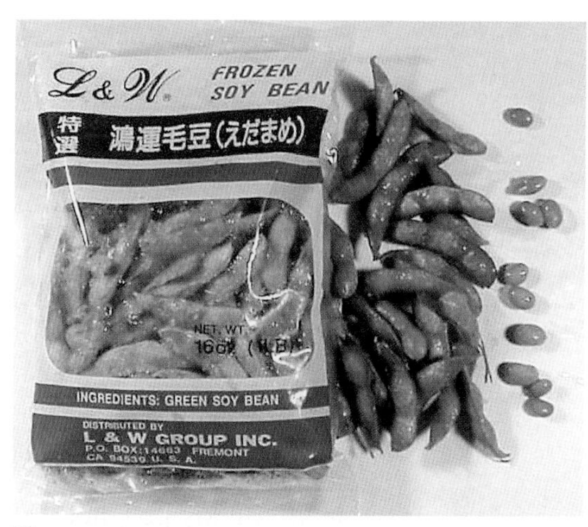

Edamame

soybeans is the best: eat the fresh bean directly and unadulterated.

Soybeans are sometimes picked when green, not yet fully mature. They are steam-cooked in the pod. You can buy them in many stores in the frozen foods section sold in one-pound bags. The Japanese call it *edamame*.

You can steam or boil the pods in salted water for a few minutes, then remove the beans from the pod, and it's just like eating peanuts. In sushi bars, edamame are often served as appetizers. If you don't feel like shelling the beans, you can buy the frozen, green soybeans already shelled. You just heat them up. The young soybeans are tender and can be eaten alone or with rice. You can also cook them with meat or vegetable dishes. They are excellent as a snack with drinks or eaten for snacks at a party. They taste good, so children easily learn to like them, especially when the parents eat the beans with the kids. Many children who have learned to eat these green soybeans like them better than cookies; my little granddaughter thinks so. If you are trying to add soy to your diet for health reasons, this can be a good alternative to drinking soy powder, which is more like a supplement than a food.

In addition to the green soybeans, there are some delicious ways to prepare mature, dried soybeans, which you can buy in health food stores as well as many grocery stores. These matured soybeans take a long time to cook and, in their whole state, are not particularly digestible. However, you can make soymilk from mature soybeans, which is a wonderful alternative to cow's milk. Soymilk is available in health food stores and large grocery chains as well, but you might be surprised how easy it is to make it yourself.

Making Soymilk

1. Soak the mature soybeans in cold water for a day. In hot weather, soak the beans in the fridge so they won't sour.
2. Drain the beans well, and bring 3 to 4 quarts of water to a boil in a separate pan.
3. Using a blender that can take the heat (stainless steel, or a plastic or glass blender preheated by filling it with

very hot tap water, letting it stand, and pouring it out), place 2 cups of beans in the blender and then add 2 cups of boiling water.

4. Purée the mixture. You can add more water for a thinner soymilk.
5. Use a large piece of unbleached muslin, clean and damp, then pour the mixture through the cloth into a bowl and squeeze the pulp that remains. Squeeze as much milk out as possible. You may need to use rubber gloves since the mixture will be very hot. It will look like beige milk. Alternatively, simply use cold water in place of boiling water. This is easier to handle, but you will get a bean like flavor in the milk. You have just made soymilk!
6. Place it in a large clean pan and bring it to a boil slowly. Simmer for a few minutes. Careful! It is rich in proteins and it can boil over easily and make a mess on the stove.
7. Add a little sugar, a dash of natural salt, and maybe a little vanilla.

You can drink this just like milk, warm or cold, or pour it over cereal in place of milk. You can also do your baking with this as a milk substitute.

You can buy commercial soymilk, but homemade is best. It looks off-white, not exactly just like milk, but homemade

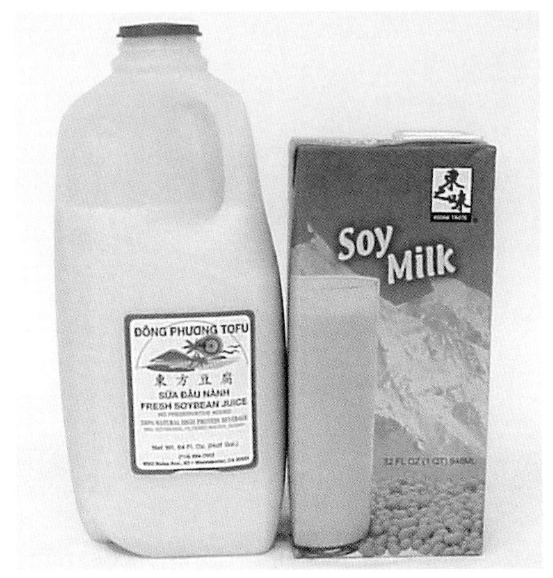

Example of commercial soymilk

and pure is what we want. Besides being fresh and very inexpensive, you can make it as rich as you like it by adjusting the amount of water in the blender. In this way, you can also make soy cream. The pulp left over after squeezing the soymilk is also good food.

In Taiwan, we used to add green onions, eggs, oil, starch, and seasonings and then make pancakes with soy pulp. Soy pancakes contain lots of protein, minerals, and vitamins, as well as fiber. However, today we have so much to eat that most people don't care to eat the soy pulp, so put it in your compost pile.

Soymilk has a unique flavor, so you'll have to get used to it if you are accustomed to cow's milk. However, if you follow the directions given here, the boiling hot water inactivates the phthalates that can give a strong, bean-like taste, and you'll find it quite palatable.

To acclimate your taste to soymilk, you can add just about anything; try chocolate soymilk or half-and-half with chocolate milk. Try soymilk when you are hungry. You may learn to like it; after all, there are a couple billion Asians that enjoy it.

Unsweetened soymilk can be used in your regular cooking and to make soups, as well. The Chinese make a popular breakfast by salting unsweetened soymilk and seasoning it with dried, small shrimp, an egg, and hot spicy oil. This is eaten with baked bread or deep-fried bread sticks.

In the Asian markets in Chinatown, both sweetened and unsweetened soymilks are available. It is much cheaper—and nicer—to make your own, but some Chinese markets do offer fresh, warm soymilk every morning. The convenience is irresistible. There is no set standard for how thick or how concentrated the soymilk is supposed to be. As you experiment with making soymilk, you can decide how concentrated you'd like your soymilk to be.

Tofu

The next step from soymilk is tofu—also called bean curd. Calcium sulfate, which is a natural mineral salt obtained

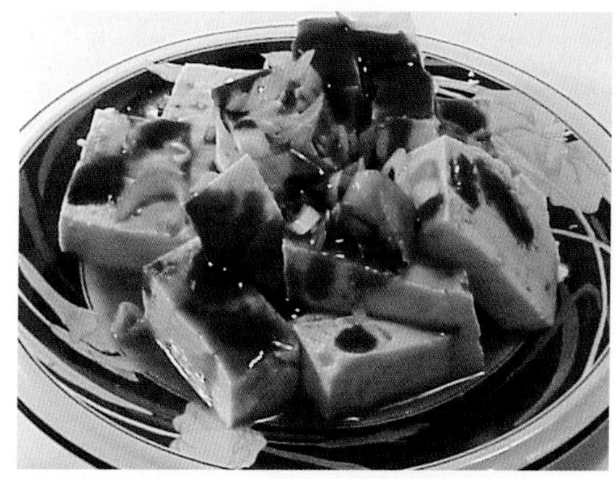

Fresh bean curd and soy sauce is a popular Taiwanese dish.

from burning a specific type of seashell and powdering it, is added to hot soymilk, which curdles it and creates a soft gelatin-like texture when the bean curd is strained and pressed.

Japanese tofu is sometimes curdled with *nigari*, which is a seawater concentrate. Tofu comes in different textures and densities; the Japanese like the soft kind, while others like it firmer. The fresh tofu can be further processed into many products, many of them made to imitate meats and fish, and it can be seasoned in countless ways. It is also preserved and fermented into even more soy products. However, around the world, fresh tofu is the most popular. In today's markets, modern packaging seals the tofu in water, which keeps it fresh for a long time when refrigerated.

The Japanese like to eat a dish made of cold tofu, called *hiyayako*. This is made by cutting tofu into one-inch cubes, seasoned only with soy sauce and with a few chopped green onions or bits of shaved dry fish. It tastes similar to cottage cheese. It can be eaten just like cottage cheese with salt and pepper. The soft Japanese tofu is better uncooked.

Because seasonings do not absorb easily into tofu, it is best to cook it slowly over medium heat to allow seasonings to penetrate the tofu slowly. Fast boiling expands the air trapped inside the tofu so it explodes; then it doesn't look—or taste—very good. Restaurants also serve deep-fried tofu, which is very tasty and popular. Deep-frying adds flavor to tofu, but don't overuse deep-fried tofu; it has too much fat.

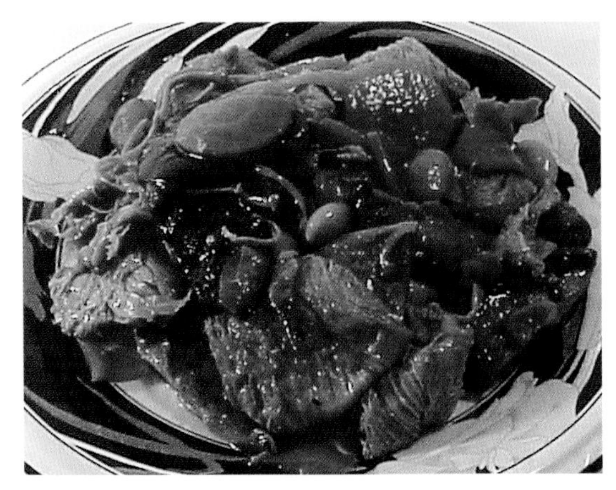

A popular bean curd dish with mushrooms and vegetables from the deli.

Bony Meats

"Don't eat too many *big* meats," the elders used to tell me. "Eat small meats and small fish instead." When they said big meats, they meant big animals like cattle and large fish, and for small meats, they meant fowl. We never knew the reason why, but it was traditional wisdom passed from generation to generation. We are starting to understand now that large predatory fish are at the top of the food chain, and their flesh contains higher concentrations of undesirable elements. Witness the recent FDA warning to pregnant women about swordfish and shark; they should avoid these foods because these sea creatures' flesh contains elevated mercury levels. I also think that we need the nutrients contained in the bones of animals, and you get those bones when you eat small animals or fish.

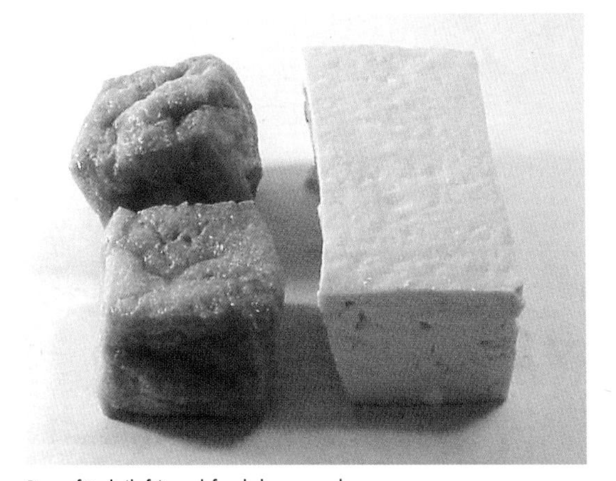

Deep fried (left) and fresh bean curd

Believe it or not, our digestive systems can digest bones easier than meat, provided you can get the bones down. The hydrochloric acid in our stomachs is very effective in digesting shells and bones. In addition, when you slow-cook the bones to make broth for soup or stew, the long cooking time soaks a rich variety of minerals from the bones that the body needs—especially for growing children.

To get these minerals, there are a few dishes popular in Asia, but relatively unknown to Americans, that incorporate the hard parts of the animal. These dishes taste good, and the Asians relish them.

Shrimp In the Shell

There is a relatively thin-shelled type of shrimp, medium-to-small in size. Chinese restaurants use this special shrimp to prepare 'pepper and salt shrimp.' It is first deep-fried, then pan-fried quickly with salt and chili peppers. The hot oil makes the thin shell crispy, while the inner meat is tender and sweet. You eat the whole thing except for the occasional hard parts. Friends from all over the world typically love this dish.

Similarly, in sushi bars, chefs typically serve *ama-ebi*, a dish where the shrimp body is prepared as *sashimi* (served raw) and the head is deep-fried and served with a sauce. The whole head is eaten, whiskers and all, except the thick shell over the head. These are two of the most popular sushi dishes, but they're difficult to make at home. The shrimp shell supplies micronutrients. Don't

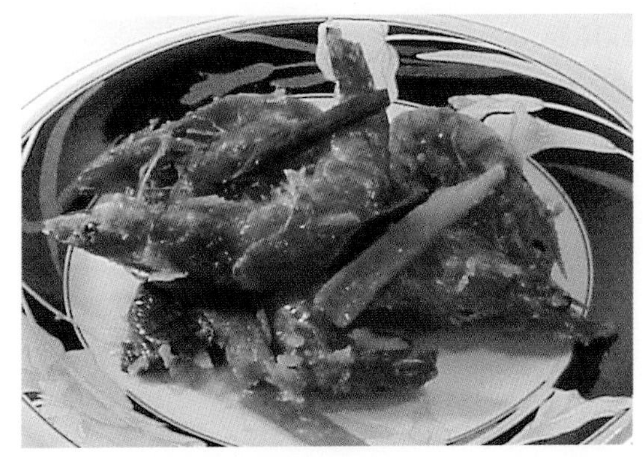

Pepper and salt shrimp dish

worry that you might not be able to digest the shell; your stomach acid easily takes care of it. In fact, most people feel very comfortable after eating *ama-ebi* because the shell acts as a natural antacid. Shrimp shells contain abundant calcium carbonate, which is the active ingredient in Tums. In the shrimp shell, we get a complete array of minerals.

Soft Shell Crab

In the Gulf coast and Atlantic Ocean, blue crabs are harvested just as they are molting and getting a new shell, which is soft for a time. At that point, they are caught and frozen. Soft shell crab is most often served deep-fried, another favorite in sushi bars. The soft shell provides many important micronutrients and minerals. Recently, Vietnam has begun exporting soft-shelled blue crabs, which are promoted as a Vietnamese delicacy. The size and quality are excellent.

Canned Seafood

You can buy all sorts of canned fish on the market today. The most familiar are sardines and tuna fish. Although most Americans prefer tuna fish, which doesn't contain the bones, canned fish such as sardines and canned salmon (with the bones included) are better for us.

In many ethnic markets, the most popular canned fish are processed with the bones. As a matter of fact, even in this country, fish containing bones are often canned, for example, sardines, anchovies, salmon, and mackerel. Most of these canned fish are well seasoned and ready to eat. The bones are well cooked, soft, and tender. They provide us with minerals and other important nutrients we need. Again, don't worry about your stomach; it can easily digest the cooked fish bones.

Seaweed

Most Asian populations eat lots of seaweed, especially in coastal areas.

It is especially popular in localities where land is scarce and the weather is cold, which makes growing vegetables difficult. Seaweeds are the vegetables of the sea; unlike vegetables nourished by sunlight, soil, and air, seaweeds are grown in the ocean, they don't take their nutrients from soil, they are nourished by sunlight and ocean water. Seaweed grows in abundance at most seashores and is rich in many important nutrients. The most popular seaweeds are dehydrated and sold in the dried food section at oriental grocery stores and health food stores.

To use dried seaweed, soak it in water for a few hours, and then stew it with meat. It takes about the same amount of time to cook seaweed tender as it does to cook meat. Properly seasoned, seaweed is delicious. The Koreans boil seaweed with chicken soup when they get a cold, or just to rejuvenate body energy. In Asian markets, you can buy ready-to-eat, cooked and seasoned seaweed, or you can buy the dried seaweed in packages to bring home and cook with meat.

If you have ever eaten sushi, you have eaten seaweed. A certain variety of seaweed, *nori*, is shredded and pressed dry in crispy thin sheets. The Japanese toast it lightly and wrap it around lightly seasoned rice, vegetables, and pickles. Koreans toast

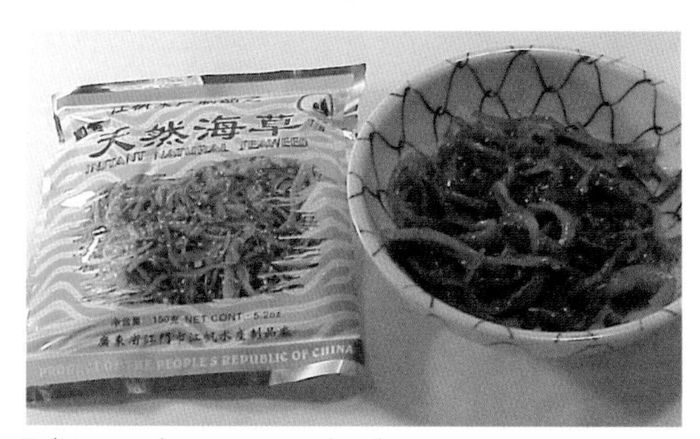

Delicious ready-to-eat seaweed package

it, cut it in small pieces, and wrap these small pieces around bites of rice. When toasted and seasoned, *nori* is packaged in snack packs, and you can eat it right out of the package. Many Americans enjoy the taste right away.

A popular, tasty Japanese seaweed is sold as a paste in small jars. It is commonly eaten with rice porridge. In addition, flakes of seaweed leaves come seasoned with sesame seeds and powdered dry fish in eight-ounce jars. You can sprinkle this over fried rice or fried noodles, and it doesn't taste fishy at all. If you like, you can sprinkle toasted, crushed *nori* over rice in the same way.

Green-Leafed Vegetables

Leafy, green veggies (and beans in the pod) contain the B vitamin folate, which is known to regulate the level of amino acid homocysteine. There is strong evidence that high blood levels of folate and a lower level of homocysteine protects us from heart disease, stroke, cancer, and Alzheimer's disease. Mothers who suffer a severe shortage of folate in their diet give birth to children with certain neurological birth defects. Recognizing the importance of folic acid, the FDA requires that many flour, rice, pasta, and grain products be fortified with folic acid. However, the exact amount we need for good health is still unknown. Therefore, it's a good idea to eat plenty of leafy, green vegetables and green beans, as discussed earlier.

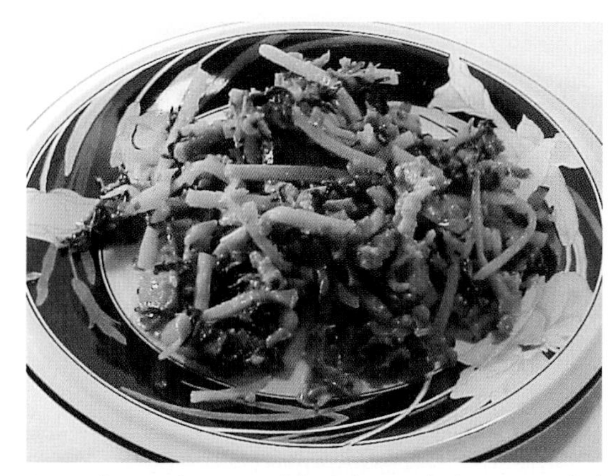

A type of mustard greens with hardy leaves; the leaves are salted to tenderize them, and then stir-fried with shredded pork and bamboo shoots. Very popular among the Taiwanese

If you don't believe in the power of micronutrients, consider the plight of the South American sloth, a slow-moving jungle animal that lives on tree leaves. In captivity, they always die prematurely even though they are fed similar tree leaves. Scientists finally figured out the problem: the leaves were harvested, cleaned, and refrigerated. In the process, the fungi and insects normally present on the leaves were removed. These provided small amounts of nutrients necessary for the sloth to survive.

Science hasn't yet identified all the micronutrients needed for humans to thrive, but I would suggest that eating a wide variety of foods is good insurance for optimal health. If you haven't learned to cook the unfamiliar foods mentioned in this book, don't worry, I'll give you some guidelines on how to do it so you can create a well-balanced, wholesome diet for you and your family. The techniques are simple enough for everyday use, and the results are delicious too.

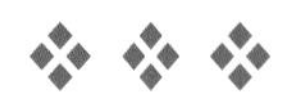

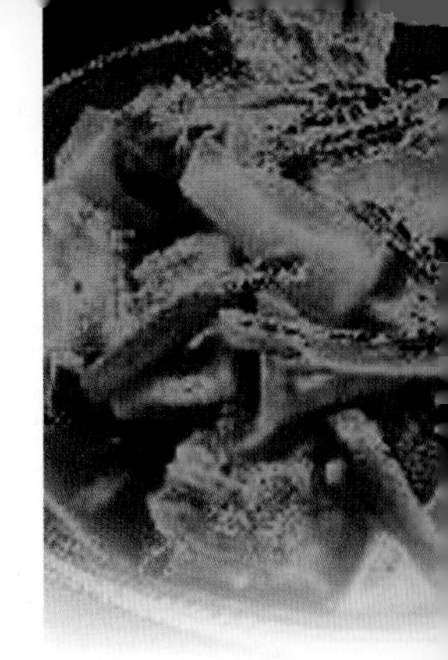

Chapter 15

Chemicals Are Hazards to Your Health

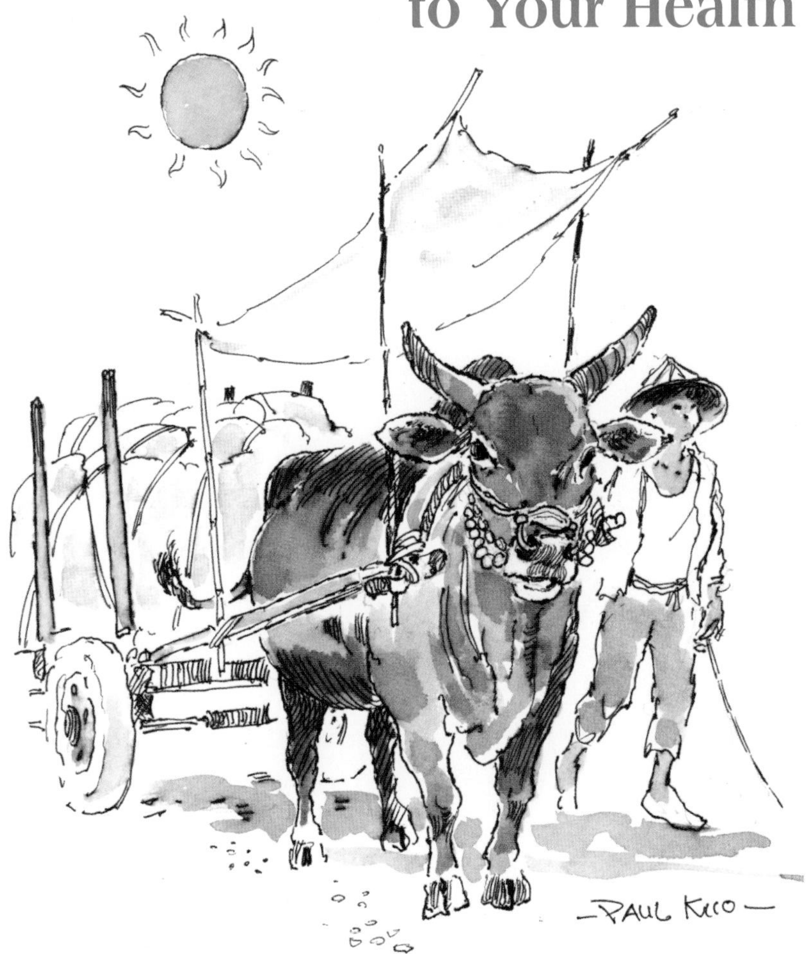

Today we know that, in addition to the foods we eat, other influences affect our health. Although I'm not writing about chemicals in this book, I want to briefly mention them here. During the last fifty years, we have come to accept that we need to live with a lot of chemicals to stay healthy. The average American household looks like a laboratory! In our kitchens, bathrooms, laundry rooms, and yards, we store an arsenal of chemicals for killing germs and insects, or just to keep clean, and most of these chemicals are harmful to our health.

Why do we use so many chemicals? We may have mistakenly bought the idea that bacteria are the enemy and must be eradicated. In reality, microorganisms are everywhere, part of a normal, natural existence. There's no way we could kill all of them, and I'm not sure it would be a good idea since our world seems to exist because of synergies between species. We keep trying to kill all the microorganisms, though, with an array of chemical products, which can eventually cause worse health problems than the bacteria we are attacking! If we want to create better health for ourselves, we can eat natural foods that build up our immunity and, at the same time, avoid the chemicals that can weaken it.

As you probably know, our bodies were designed to handle bacterial and viral invasion. When we are exposed to harmful bacteria and viruses, our immune systems go into action to generate antibodies to fight the invaders. We retain these antibodies and they help us fight subsequent infections. Immunizations work on the same principle. The more germs you're exposed to, the more types of antibodies your body will produce. If you are exposed to unfamiliar germs, your body sometimes takes a while to adjust. That's why travelers, for example, sometimes get diarrhea, because their bodies can't yet handle the bacteria in the foreign country's water.

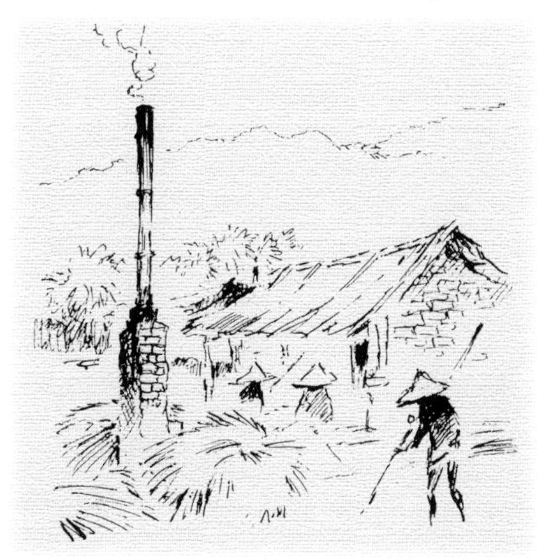

Mosquito beware. Citronella oil, a Taiwan export, is distilled from special grasses grown on Taiwan mountainsides. Industry finds many uses for this oil; it may even end up in my lady's perfume.

Of course, I'm not suggesting that we don't keep clean! I am recommending, however, that we become more aware of the bad effects of chemicals on our health and that we don't become so obsessed with chemical solutions. Our bodies naturally produce antibodies against disease, but we can't produce antibodies for chemical toxicity. We absorb chemicals through the skin, and also by eating and breathing them. Chemicals kill germs, which may even deprive our bodies of the opportunity to make antibodies against them.

Chemicals not only cause cell damage, but also many pesticides mimic hormones, particularly estrogen, which can cause abnormal cell growth leading to cancer. Continued exposure to chemicals—even in low

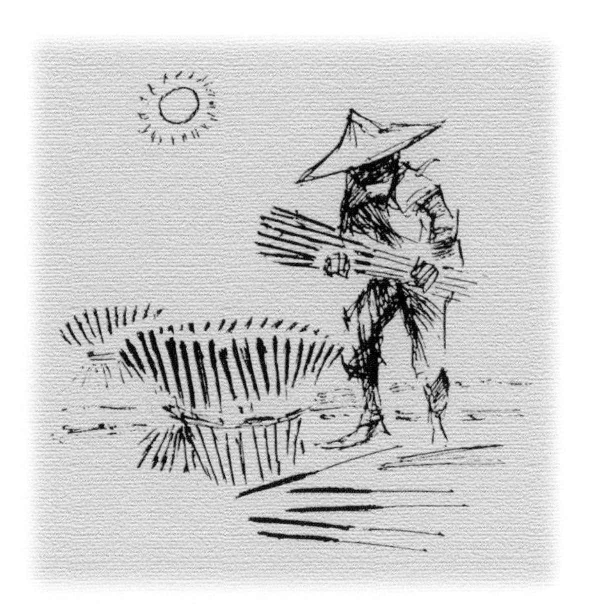

Symbol of worship. The annual consumption of joss sticks in Taiwan must reach astronomical figures. Their main purpose is for worship in temple and shrine. However, the burning punk is sometimes used to repel mosquitoes or substitute for a bicycle light.

doses—in the long run will weaken our immunity. This, in itself, might have much to do with the widespread immune-system disorders we suffer with today. We may have a difficult time pinpointing the exact reason for our health problems, but I am convinced that the chemicals we use are a big part of the problem.

What to do? You can take a look at the chemicals you use in your home and yard and eliminate what you can. There are natural home care products available which are not toxic. Don't worry if you find a few insects in your home; insects are harmless, for the most part, but insecticides are dangerous. If you just can't stand having that spider in the family room, have somebody take him outside. I observed first-hand in Taiwan what insecticides could do when the American government, as part of the economic aid program, sprayed my entire village with DDT against mosquitoes. It killed the mosquitoes, as well as most of the cats and small animals. And ironically, the mosquitoes were gone for a while, but returned with a vengeance a few months later.

Even if you keep everybody away when you spray for insects, you need to know that all materials absorb the chemicals including cabinets, counter tops, furniture, drapes, walls, and ceilings. If you absolutely must fumigate for insects, after spraying, heat your house as warm as possible, and ventilate it for a day or two, then cool it down before you move back in. Warm surfaces retain less chemical molecules. Personally, as a scientist, knowing the toxicity of the chemicals and how they can damage the body, I'd rather put up with a few insects than risk using pesticides inside the house. Pesticides may linger in the house in low concentrations for a very long time; although conventional detection devices can't find them, they are still there.

People who suffer immune deficiency diseases are often surprised to see how much they improve when they eliminate chemicals from their lives. It's a good idea to use as few as possible for optimal health. Wash or rinse with plenty of hot water to get things clean and sanitary. Chlorinated water and a high enough temperature will kill most harmful bacteria or germs without other chemicals.

It's a worthy goal to move toward a simpler, more natural lifestyle. It is my hope that you will enjoy reading this book, and that it will empower you to adapt your lifestyle to a new way of eating—and living—that can bring you good health for the rest of a long life.

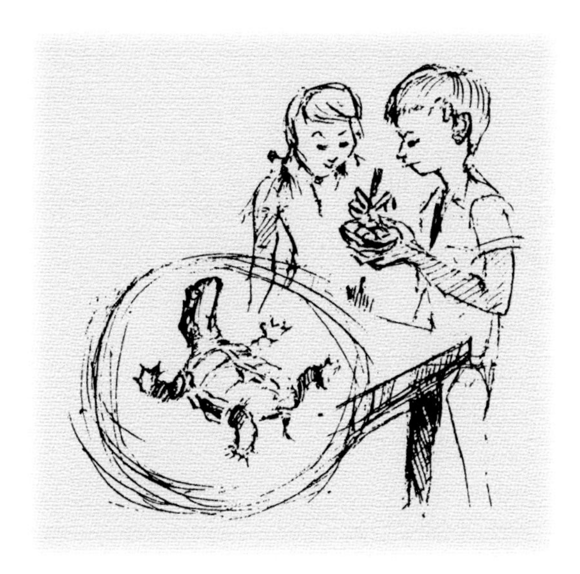

Sin offering. In order to make reparation for an evil deed, the offender marks his name on the back of a turtle and sets it free. The turtle lives for a legendary 10,000 years piling up merit for the one who saved its life.

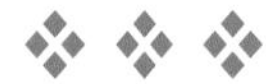

INDEX

T